BUTTERFLY SPIRIT

CHECK OUT ALL MY BOOKS!

BUTTERFLY SPIRIT

THIS BOOK BELONGS TO:

____

NAME

____

DATE & TIME

____

SIGNATURE

BUTTERFLY SPIRIT

BUTTERFLY SPIRIT

BUTTERFLY SPIRIT

This page belongs to the readers who dare to dream and take action. Each word is a gentle reminder that within you lies the power to manifest your desires and transform your reality. This is your space to reflect, grow, and create the life you envision. Use these pages to write your story and embrace the beautiful journey of becoming.

BUTTERFLY SPIRIT

Dedication

This book is dedicated to GOD our creator, all the dreamers, seekers, and believers who are ready to transform their lives.

those who dare to embrace change, trust in their journey, and illuminate the world with their unique light.

May you always remember that you are worthy of your desires and capable of achieving your greatest dreams.

BUTTERFLY SPIRIT

Introduction

Welcome to S.Petit , a journey of transformation and self-discovery guided by the wisdom of the Butterfly Spirit. In a world that often feels overwhelming, it is essential to remember that change is not only possible; it is a natural part of life.

Much like a butterfly emerging from its chrysalis, we, too, can break free from our limitations and embrace the beauty that lies within us.

This book is designed to help you unlock your potential and manifest your desires. Through practical exercises, heartfelt reflections, and powerful affirmations, you will learn to cultivate a mindset that attracts abundance, joy, and success. Each chapter invites you to explore different facets of your life, encouraging you to embrace the changes you wish to see.

As you navigate these pages, I encourage you to approach this journey with an open heart and mind. Allow yourself to be vulnerable, to dream big, and to trust the process of transformation. Your Butterfly Spirit is waiting to soar!

BUTTERFLY SPIRIT

Action Steps
(Identify actionable steps you can take this week to support your manifestation.)
What will I do this week to move closer to my desires?

----

7. Closing Intention
(Conclude your ritual with a closing statement.)
"Thank you, Universe, for the guidance and support. I trust that my desires are manifesting in divine timing. I am ready to receive all the blessings that come my way. So it is, and so it shall be."

8. Follow-Up Journal Entry
(After your ritual, write a follow-up entry about your feelings and insights.)
How did this ritual make me feel?

What did I learn about my desires?

Tips for Success
Consistency: Perform this ritual weekly to strengthen your manifestation practice.
Stay Open: Be receptive to the signs and opportunities that come your way.
Positive Mindset: Maintain a positive outlook throughout the week to attract your desires.

BUTTERFLY SPIRIT

PRAYER TO GOD
FOR
TRANSFORMATION AND PROSPERITY

Dear Heavenly Father,
I come before You with a humble and open heart, seeking Your
divine guidance and blessings in my life. I trust in Your power
to transform me, to shape me into the person You have
called me to be. Just as the butterfly emerges from its
chrysalis, I ask for Your strength to break free from all that
holds me back.

Lord, guide me through the changes I must make, and help me
embrace each season of growth. Let me not fear the unknown,
but trust that You are with me, molding my spirit with grace
and purpose. Fill my heart with the courage to pursue the
dreams You have placed within me.
As I walk this path of transformation, I pray for prosperity—
not just in material wealth, but in wisdom, love, and spiritual
abundance. Bless the work of my hands and the desires of
my heart, and allow me to prosper in ways that reflect Your
glory.

Help me to always remember that true prosperity begins with
a soul rooted in Your love. Guide me to make wise decisions,
to live with integrity, and to honor You in all that I do. May
Your light shine through me, leading me toward success and
fulfillment in all areas of my life.
Thank You, Lord, for Your everlasting love, for Your provision,
and for the transformation You are bringing into my life. I
trust in Your plan, knowing that with You, all things are
possible.
In Your Holy Name, I pray.
Amen.

BUTTERFLY SPIRIT

Butterflies inspire growth through their powerful symbolism of transformation, resilience, and beauty, which resonates deeply with the human experience.

Here are several ways they inspire personal growth:

The butterfly's delicate yet powerful presence reminds us that growth requires change, courage, and trust in the process.

BUTTERFLY SPIRIT

Letting Go of the Old:

A caterpillar must shed its old form to become a butterfly, which reflects the need to let go of outdated mindsets, habits, or limitations. In our own lives, personal growth often requires releasing the past to make room for new opportunities.

Freedom and Expansion:

Once the butterfly emerges, it tak
es flight with grace and freedom, symbolizing how growth leads to expansion—new perspectives, experiences, and freedom to explore our full potential. This inspires us to spread our wings and embrace life's opportunities without fear.

Beauty in Diversity:

Butterflies come in countless colors and patterns, reminding us that growth doesn't have a single form. Each person's journey is unique, and there is beauty in diversity, both in nature and in personal development.

Living in the Moment: Butterflies have relatively short lifespans, yet they live fully in each moment. This inspires growth by encouraging us to focus on the present, savor life's beauty, and make the most of every opportunity for learning and development.

BUTTERFLY SPIRIT

Symbol of Transformation

The butterfly's life cycle—moving from egg to caterpillar, then chrysalis, and finally emerging as a butterfly—mirrors our own capacity for transformation. It teaches that growth often requires change, even when it's difficult or uncomfortable.

Like the butterfly, we must sometimes undergo periods of uncertainty or hardship (the chrysalis stage) before we emerge stronger and more beautiful.

Embracing Change:

Butterflies show that change is a natural part of life and can lead to profound beauty. Their metamorphosis encourages us to embrace transitions rather than fear them, knowing that change is a pathway to becoming the best version of ourselves.

Resilience and Patience:

The butterfly's journey requires patience, as each stage takes time. This reminds us that growth is a process, not an overnight event. It encourages perseverance, teaching us to trust the process even when we can't see immediate results.

BUTTERFLY SPIRIT

She has long, flowing hair that cascades down her back like a shimmering waterfall, catching the light with every movement. Her hair is not just an accessory; it is a reflection of her vibrant personality—perhaps a rich, warm hue that complements her complexion or a bold color that makes her stand out in any crowd. Her pretty skin glows with a radiant quality, reflecting her commitment to self-care and wellness.

Her look is a vital part of her identity; she takes pride in how she presents herself to the world. Whether she's adorned in chic outfits that enhance her figure or sporting casual attire that exudes effortless elegance, every detail is carefully considered. She understands the power of beauty, not just as a superficial trait but as a way to express her confidence and individuality.

Her gaze is captivating, framed by long lashes and perfectly shaped brows that draw attention to her expressive eyes—perhaps a striking color that tells its own story. She carries herself with grace and poise, embodying an aura of charm and allure that leaves a lasting impression on everyone she meets.

BUTTERFLY SPIRIT

Butterfly Spirit's Backstory

Butterfly Spirit was once a mortal woman, living in a world filled with uncertainty and challenges. She was known for her compassion, ambition, and beauty, but her life was not easy.

From an early age, she faced adversity, constantly forced to adapt and transform in the face of hardship. Each time she encountered obstacles, she found a way to rise above them, reinventing herself and growing stronger.

Her defining moment came during a period of deep personal crisis. Struggling with loss and the fear of failure, she was visited by a mysterious cosmic force—a being of pure light and energy.

This being revealed to her the secret of continuous transformation, showing her that life is a cycle of death and rebirth and that every ending is a new beginning. The cosmic force merged with her, imbuing her with the power to constantly evolve, like a butterfly emerging from a chrysalis. From that moment on, she became Butterfly Spirit, a symbol of growth, beauty, and limitless potential.

Her journey is one of self-discovery, as she learns to master the ability to shed old versions of herself and step into her full power. Along the way, she helps others unlock their own potential, guiding them toward personal growth and transformation.

BUTTERFLY SPIRIT

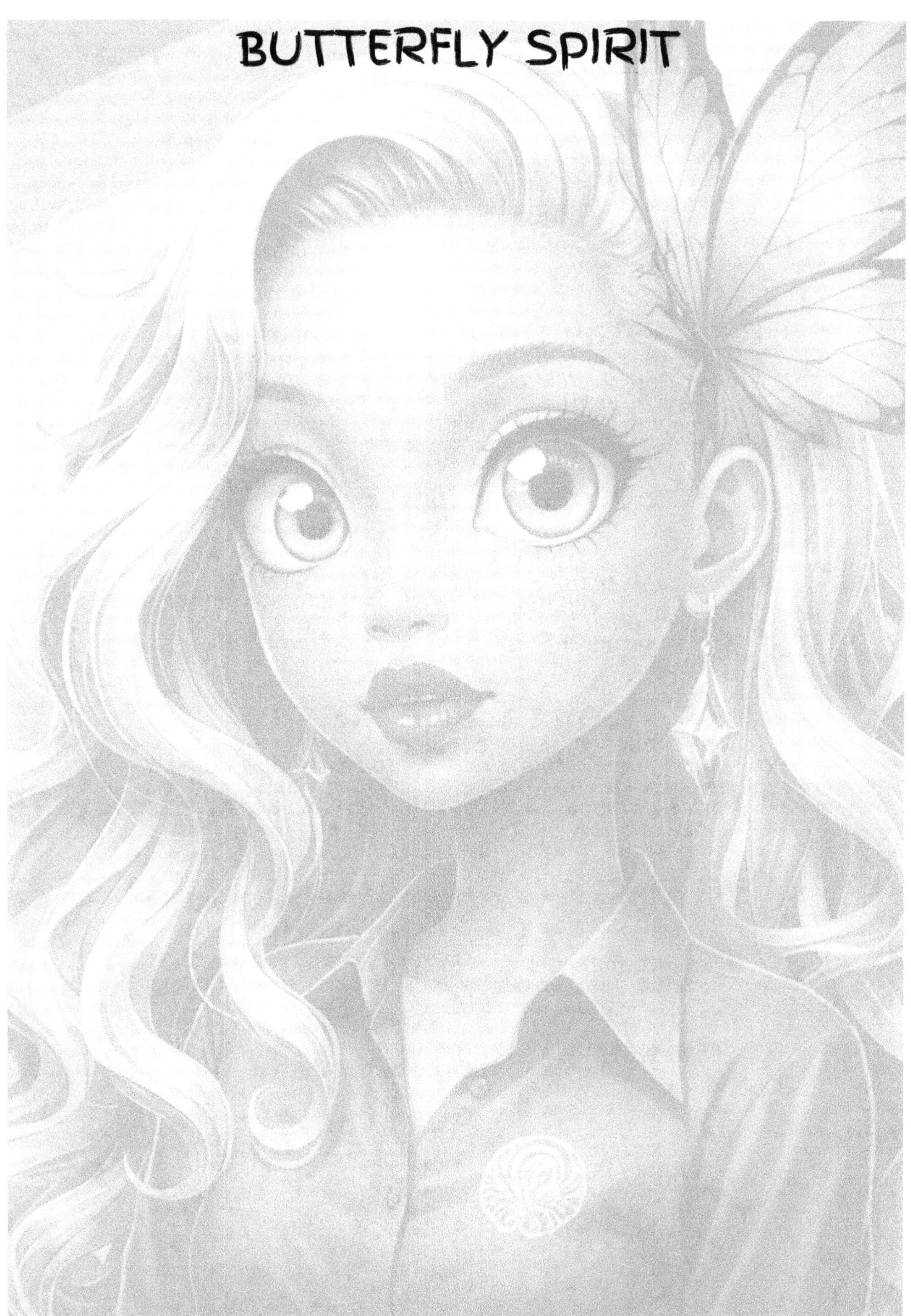

BUTTERFLY SPIRIT

Stay Open to Learning

Growth thrives on curiosity and the willingness to learn. Maintain a growth mindset by embracing new experiences, ideas, and skills. Take courses, read books, seek feedback, or engage with diverse perspectives to keep expanding your knowledge.

Surround Yourself with Positive Influences

The people around you significantly impact your ability to maintain growth. Surround yourself with individuals who inspire, challenge, and support your development. These could be mentors, peers, or communities that share your values and encourage your continued evolution.

Embrace Challenges

View challenges as opportunities for further growth. When faced with difficulties, focus on how they can help you develop resilience, problem-solving skills, or new perspectives. Growth often occurs outside of your comfort zone, so don't shy away from obstacles.

Practice Consistency and Discipline

Maintaining growth requires consistent effort. Develop daily or weekly habits that reinforce your progress, whether it's exercising, practicing mindfulness, or working toward your goals. Consistency builds momentum and keeps you from slipping back into old patterns.

Stay Adaptable

Growth is a continuous process, and life will inevitably bring changes. Be adaptable and open to shifting your path when needed. Flexibility ensures you can maintain progress even when faced with unexpected circumstances or when new opportunities arise.

BUTTERFLY SPIRIT

Celebrate Progress

Acknowledge and celebrate your achievements, no matter how small. Recognizing your wins reinforces your growth mindset and boosts motivation to continue. It also helps you appreciate the journey, not just the destination.

Take Care of Your Well-Being

Physical, mental, and emotional well-being are essential for sustaining growth. Make self-care a priority—maintain a healthy lifestyle, manage stress, and ensure you get enough rest. A balanced mind and body provide the energy and clarity needed for continuous improvement.

Remain Humble and Grateful

Stay humble about your progress and remain grateful for the lessons learned along the way. Gratitude fosters a positive mindset and reminds you that growth is a privilege, not just an obligation. It helps you remain grounded and open to learning from every experience.

Be Patient and Persistent

Growth takes time, so be patient with yourself during the process. Not every step will be smooth, and there will be setbacks. Persistence is key—view setbacks as learning opportunities rather than failures and continue pushing forward with determination.

Engage in Mindfulness or Meditation

Mindfulness practices can help you stay present, focused, and aware of your growth journey. Meditation, deep breathing, or even simple mindfulness exercises can help you remain centered, making it easier to maintain personal development over the long term.

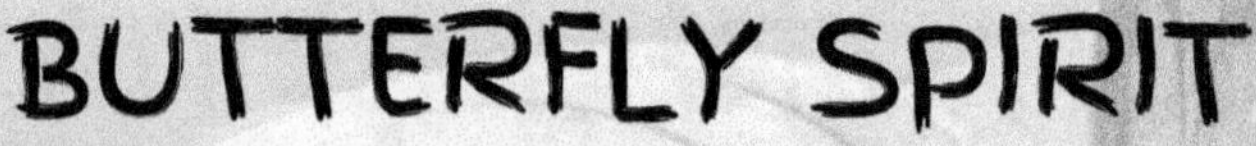

BUTTERFLY SPIRIT

Maintaining growth is an ongoing process that requires intentionality, resilience, and a lifelong commitment to bettering yourself.

By cultivating these habits and mindsets, you can ensure that personal growth becomes a continuous and rewarding part of your life.

BUTTERFLY SPIRIT

Expressing beauty is a multifaceted endeavor that encompasses not just physical appearance but also inner qualities and how you carry yourself in the world.

Here are several ways to express beauty holistically:

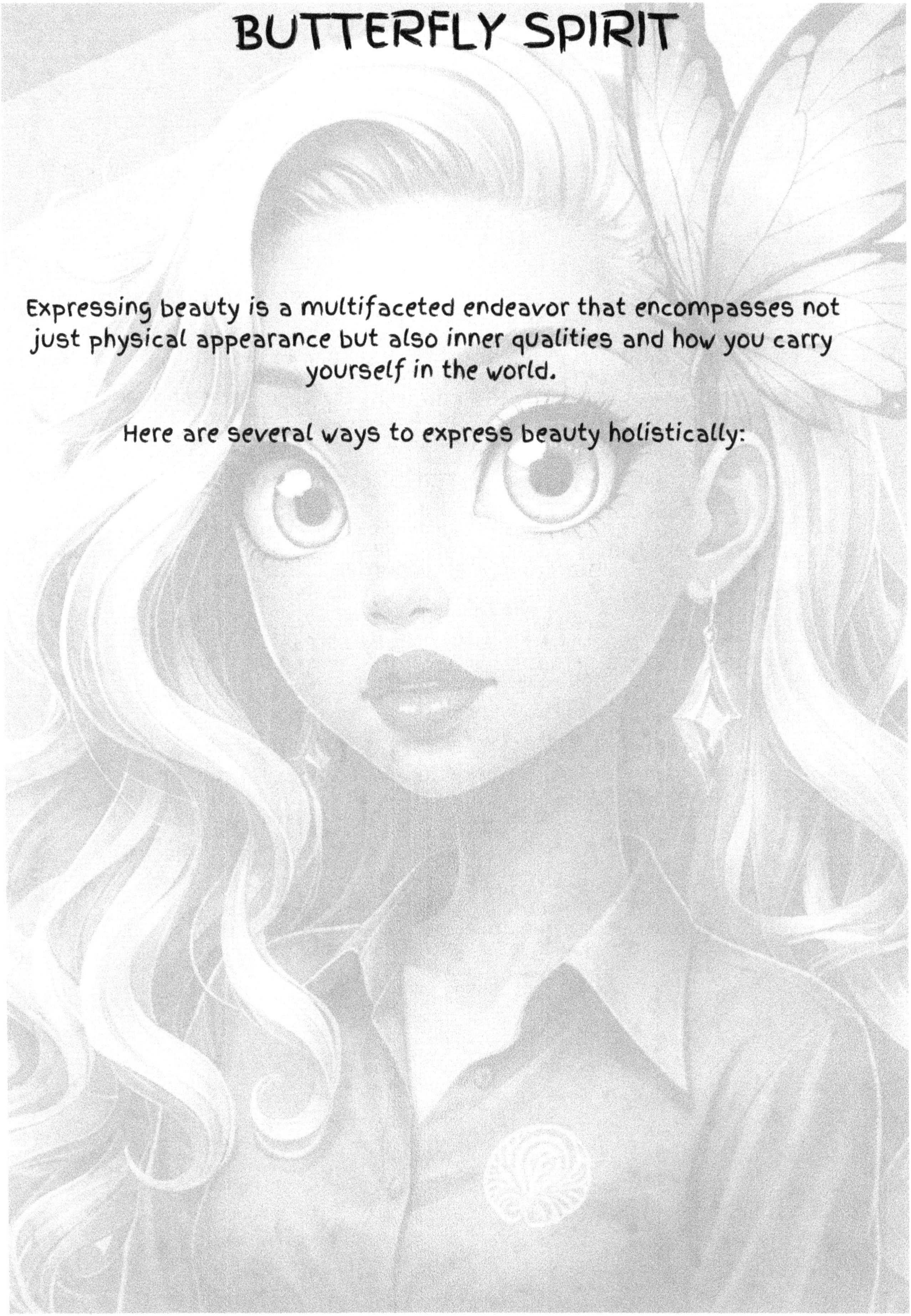

BUTTERFLY SPIRIT

Body Language

Posture: Stand tall with confidence. Good posture not only enhances your appearance but also communicates confidence and self-assuredness.
Smiling: A genuine smile can light up your face and create warmth. It's one of the simplest yet most powerful ways to express beauty.

Nurture Inner Beauty

Kindness and Compassion: Treat others with kindness and empathy. Your inner beauty shines when you foster positive relationships and create a supportive environment.

Authenticity:

Be true to yourself. Authenticity attracts others and fosters genuine connections, enhancing your beauty from within.

Mindfulness and Presence

Be Present: Practice mindfulness to appreciate the moment, Being fully present can enhance your interactions and allow your natural beauty to emerge.

Gratitude:

Cultivate a mindset of gratitude for your body, appearance, and abilities. Gratitude fosters positivity and radiates beauty.

BUTTERFLY SPIRIT

Cultivate Confidence

Self-Acceptance: Embrace who you are, including your flaws and imperfections. Confidence shines through when you accept and love yourself as you are.

Positive Self-Talk:

Use affirmations and positive language when thinking about or speaking to yourself. This helps to build a healthy self-image.

Grooming and Personal Care

Skincare: Invest time in a skincare routine that nourishes and enhances your natural glow. Healthy, radiant skin often reflects inner well-being.
Hairstyling: Experiment with hairstyles that complement your features. Whether you prefer it sleek, curly, or colorful, how you style your hair can express your personality.

Fashion Choices

Dress to Express: Wear clothes that make you feel good and reflect your personality. The right outfit can enhance your confidence and convey your unique style.

Accessorizing:

Use accessories like jewelry, scarves, or hats to add flair to your look.
Thoughtful accessories can showcase your individuality and taste.

BUTTERFLY SPIRIT

Engage with Nature

Outdoor Activities: Spend time in nature, whether through hiking, gardening, or simply enjoying the outdoors. Nature can inspire a sense of beauty and tranquility that reflects in your demeanor.

Natural Elements:

Incorporate natural materials and themes into your life—like plants in your home, earthy colors in your wardrobe, or natural makeup looks.

Self-Expression Through Art

Photography: Capture moments of beauty in everyday life. This can help you appreciate the beauty around you and in yourself.

Writing:

Express your thoughts and feelings through poetry or prose. Writing can articulate your inner beauty and resonate with others.

Mindful Beauty Practices

Meditation:

Practice mindfulness or meditation to connect with your inner self. This can enhance your sense of peace and beauty from within.

Affirmative Practices:

Incorporate beauty affirmations into your daily routine to reinforce a positive self-image.

BUTTERFLY SPIRIT

Creative Expression

Artistic Outlets: Explore painting, writing, dancing, or any form of creative expression. Engaging in the arts can help you connect with your inner beauty and share it with the world.

Personal Projects:

Work on projects that excite you or align with your passions. This not only nurtures your inner beauty but also showcases your talents.

Healthy Lifestyle

Nutrition: Nourish your body with wholesome foods that promote health and vitality. A balanced diet can enhance your natural beauty and energy levels.
Exercise: Engage in physical activity that you enjoy. Exercise boosts endorphins, promotes confidence, and contributes to a healthy appearance.

Cultivate Positive Relationships

Surround Yourself with Supportive People: Build a circle of friends and family who uplift you. Positive relationships enhance your sense of self-worth and radiate beauty.

Compliments and Affirmations:

Share genuine compliments with others and accept them graciously. This fosters a positive atmosphere and enhances everyone's sense of beauty.

BUTTERFLY SPIRIT

Ultimately, expressing beauty is about embracing who you are—inside and out. It's an ongoing journey that involves self-discovery, self-care, and authenticity.

By focusing on both inner and outer qualities, you can cultivate a beauty that resonates with others and reflects your true self.

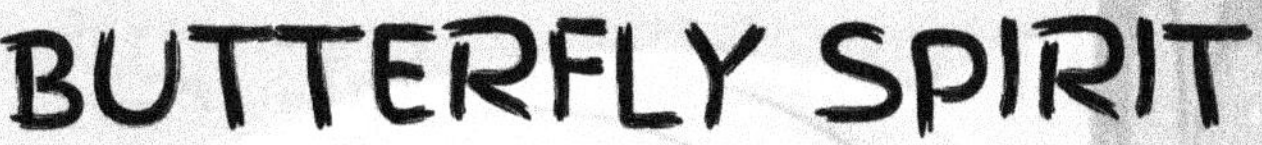

BUTTERFLY SPIRIT

Here's a comprehensive beauty routine to help you maintain a healthy, radiant appearance, covering skincare, makeup, hair care, and overall wellness.

BUTTERFLY SPIRIT

Cleansing
Frequency: Cleanse your face twice a day—once in the morning and once before bed.
Product Type: Use a gentle cleanser suited to your skin type (gel for oily skin, cream for dry skin, etc.).

Exfoliation
Frequency: Exfoliate 1-2 times a week to remove dead skin cells and promote cell turnover.
Method: Use physical exfoliants (scrubs) or chemical exfoliants (AHA/BHA) based on your skin's needs.

Toning
Purpose: Toners help to balance your skin's pH and remove any leftover impurities.
Ingredients: Look for hydrating ingredients like rose water or soothing ingredients like witch hazel.

Moisturizing
Frequency: Moisturize daily, after cleansing and toning.
Product Type: Choose a lightweight gel moisturizer for oily skin or a thicker cream for dry skin.

Sun Protection
Frequency: Apply sunscreen every morning, even on cloudy days.

SPF: Use a broad-spectrum sunscreen with at least SPF 30, and reapply every two hours if outdoors.

BUTTERFLY SPIRIT

Special Treatments

Serums: Incorporate serums with active ingredients (like Vitamin C for brightness or hyaluronic acid for hydration) based on your skin concerns.

Masks:

Use a face mask once a week for added hydration or treatment.
Makeup Routine

Prep Your Skin

Primer: Use a makeup primer to create a smooth base for your foundation and help it last longer.

Foundation

Type: Choose a foundation type that suits your skin type (liquid, cream, powder).
Application: Use a makeup sponge or brush for an even application.

Concealer

Purpose: Apply concealer to cover blemishes, dark circles, or redness.

Technique:

Use a light hand and blend well for a natural finish.

BUTTERFLY SPIRIT

Blush and Bronzer

Blush: Apply blush to the apples of your cheeks for a healthy glow.

Bronzer: Use bronzer to add warmth and definition to your face.

Eyes

Eyeshadow: Use neutral tones for everyday looks, and don't hesitate to play with colors for special occasions.

Eyeliner and Mascara:

Define your eyes with eyeliner and add volume to your lashes with mascara.

Brows

Shaping: Keep your brows well-groomed. Fill in any sparse areas with a brow pencil or powder.

Lips

Hydration: Exfoliate and moisturize your lips before applying lipstick or gloss.

Color:

Choose lip colors that enhance your natural beauty, whether a subtle nude or a bold red.

BUTTERFLY SPIRIT

Hair Care Routine

Cleansing

Frequency: Wash your hair 2-3 times a week, or as needed based on your hair type.

Shampoo: Use a sulfate-free shampoo to maintain moisture.

Conditioning

Conditioner: Always use a conditioner after shampooing to hydrate and detangle your hair.

Deep Conditioning:

Use a deep conditioner or hair mask once a week for extra hydration.

Styling

Heat Protection: Always apply a heat protectant before using heat styling tools.

Limit Heat:

Try to limit the use of heat styling tools to prevent damage.

Regular Trims

Frequency: Trim your hair every 6-8 weeks to maintain healthy ends and prevent split ends.

BUTTERFLY SPIRIT

Creating a personalized beauty routine that incorporates these elements can help you express and maintain your beauty. Remember that consistency is key; results take time, so be patient with yourself as you work towards your beauty goals! Adjust these tips based on your unique skin type, hair type, and lifestyle for the best results.

As a human butterfly spirit, she embodies qualities and powers that reflect the transformative and ethereal nature of butterflies.

Here are some powers and attributes she might possess:

BUTTERFLY SPIRIT

Transformation

Metamorphosis: She has the ability to undergo personal transformations, adapting to different situations and evolving into her best self, much like a butterfly changes through its life stages.

Healing

Emotional Healing: She possesses the power to heal emotional wounds in herself and others, bringing comfort and encouragement through her kind and nurturing presence.

Physical Healing:

She may have the ability to heal minor injuries or ailments, spreading vitality and wellness wherever she goes.

Empathy and Intuition

Deep Empathy: She can sense the emotions and needs of those around her, helping her connect with others on a profound level.

Intuitive Insights:

Her intuition guides her decisions and helps her navigate life's challenges, making her a wise and insightful companion.

Beauty and Charm

Enchanting Presence: She radiates beauty and charm, drawing people in with her magnetic energy. Her presence uplifts those around her, fostering a sense of joy and inspiration.

Aura of Attraction:

Her ethereal quality allows her to attract positivity and abundance into her life and the lives of others.

BUTTERFLY SPIRIT

Flight and Freedom

Flight: She can float or glide gracefully, symbolizing freedom and liberation. This power allows her to rise above challenges and gain a new perspective on life.

Escape from Constraints:

She can navigate and escape situations that feel limiting or confining, embodying the spirit of freedom.

Connection to Nature

Nature Communication: She can communicate with animals and plants, fostering a deep connection with nature and its rhythms.
Elemental Affinity: She may have powers related to the elements, such as the ability to summon gentle breezes or encourage flowers to bloom.

Wisdom and Guidance

Mentorship: She possesses the wisdom gained from her experiences and can guide others through their transformations and challenges.
Visionary Thinking: Her insights often inspire others to see the bigger picture and embrace change in their own lives.

Joy and Playfulness

Spreading Joy: Her laughter and playful spirit bring joy to those around her, reminding others of the beauty and lightness of life.

Creative Expression:

She has a natural talent for creativity, whether through art, music, or dance, allowing her to express her emotions and inspire others.

Resilience and Strength

Inner Strength: Despite her delicate appearance, she possesses great resilience and strength, overcoming challenges with grace and determination.

Adaptability:

She can adapt to changing circumstances, embracing new beginnings and opportunities with an open heart.

BUTTERFLY SPIRIT

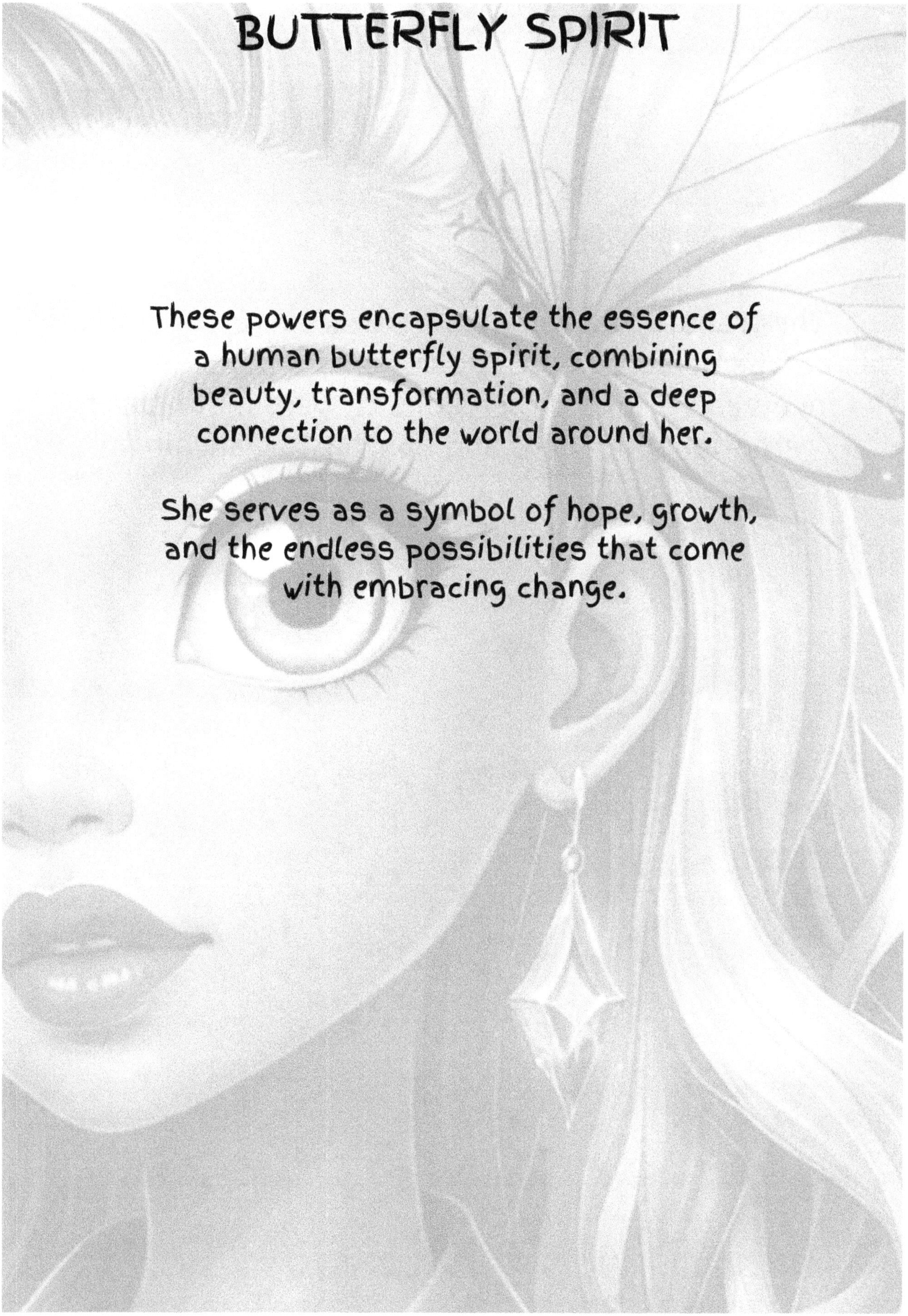

These powers encapsulate the essence of
a human butterfly spirit, combining
beauty, transformation, and a deep
connection to the world around her.

She serves as a symbol of hope, growth,
and the endless possibilities that come
with embracing change.

BUTTERFLY SPIRIT

The transformation of a human butterfly spirit can be depicted as a multi-layered process that involves various dimensions of personal growth, emotional healing, and spiritual awakening.

Here's how she might transform:

BUTTERFLY SPIRIT

Embracing Spirituality

Connecting with Nature: Spending time in nature rejuvenates her spirit and helps her feel more connected to the world around her. Nature serves as a constant reminder of the cycles of transformation.

Meditation and Rituals: Engaging in spiritual practices, such as meditation or rituals, enables her to tap into her inner wisdom and gain insights about her path.

Expressing Creativity

Artistic Outlets: She channels her emotions into creative pursuits like painting, writing, or dancing, allowing her to express her evolving self and share her journey with others.

Manifestation: Through visualization and affirmations, she manifests her dreams, shaping her reality and reinforcing her transformation.

Developing Resilience

Facing Adversity: When faced with setbacks, she learns to view them as opportunities for growth, cultivating resilience and strength.

Positive Mindset: By focusing on gratitude and maintaining a positive outlook, she nurtures her mental and emotional well-being during her transformation.

BUTTERFLY SPIRIT

As a human butterfly spirit, she embodies qualities and powers that reflect the transformative and ethereal nature of butterflies.

Here are some powers and attributes she might possess:

Manifestation

Manifesting Dreams: She has the ability to manifest her desires and dreams through focused intention and visualization, creating positive change in her life and the lives of others.

BUTTERFLY SPIRIT

Transformation

Metamorphosis: She can undergo personal transformations, adapting to different situations and evolving into her best self, much like a butterfly changes through its life stages.

Healing

Emotional Healing: She possesses the power to heal emotional wounds in herself and others, bringing comfort and encouragement through her kind and nurturing presence.

Physical Healing: She may have the ability to heal minor injuries or ailments, spreading vitality and wellness wherever she goes.

Empathy and Intuition

Deep Empathy: She can sense the emotions and needs of those around her, helping her connect with others on a profound level.

Intuitive Insights: Her intuition guides her decisions and helps her navigate life's challenges, making her a wise and insightful companion.

BUTTERFLY SPIRIT

Beauty and Charm

Enchanting Presence: She radiates beauty and charm, drawing people in with her magnetic energy. Her presence uplifts those around her, fostering a sense of joy and inspiration.

Aura of Attraction: Her ethereal quality allows her to attract positivity and abundance into her life and the lives of others.

Flight and Freedom

Flight: She has the ability to float or glide gracefully, symbolizing freedom and liberation. This power allows her to rise above challenges and gain a new perspective on life.

Escape from Constraints: She can navigate and escape situations that feel limiting or confining, embodying the spirit of freedom.

Connection to Nature

Nature Communication: She has the ability to communicate with animals and plants, fostering a deep connection with nature and its rhythms.

Elemental Affinity: She may have powers related to the elements, such as the ability to summon gentle breezes or encourage flowers to bloom.

BUTTERFLY SPIRIT

Wisdom and Guidance

Mentorship: She possesses the wisdom gained from her experiences and is able to guide others through their transformations and challenges.
Visionary Thinking: Her insights often inspire others to see the bigger picture and embrace change in their own lives.

Joy and Playfulness

Spreading Joy: Her laughter and playful spirit bring joy to those around her, reminding others of the beauty and lightness of life.
Creative Expression: She has a natural talent for creativity, whether through art, music, or dance, allowing her to express her emotions and inspire others.

Resilience and Strength

Inner Strength: Despite her delicate appearance, she possesses great resilience and strength, overcoming challenges with grace and determination.
Adaptability: She can adapt to changing circumstances, embracing new beginnings and opportunities with an open heart.

BUTTERFLY SPIRIT

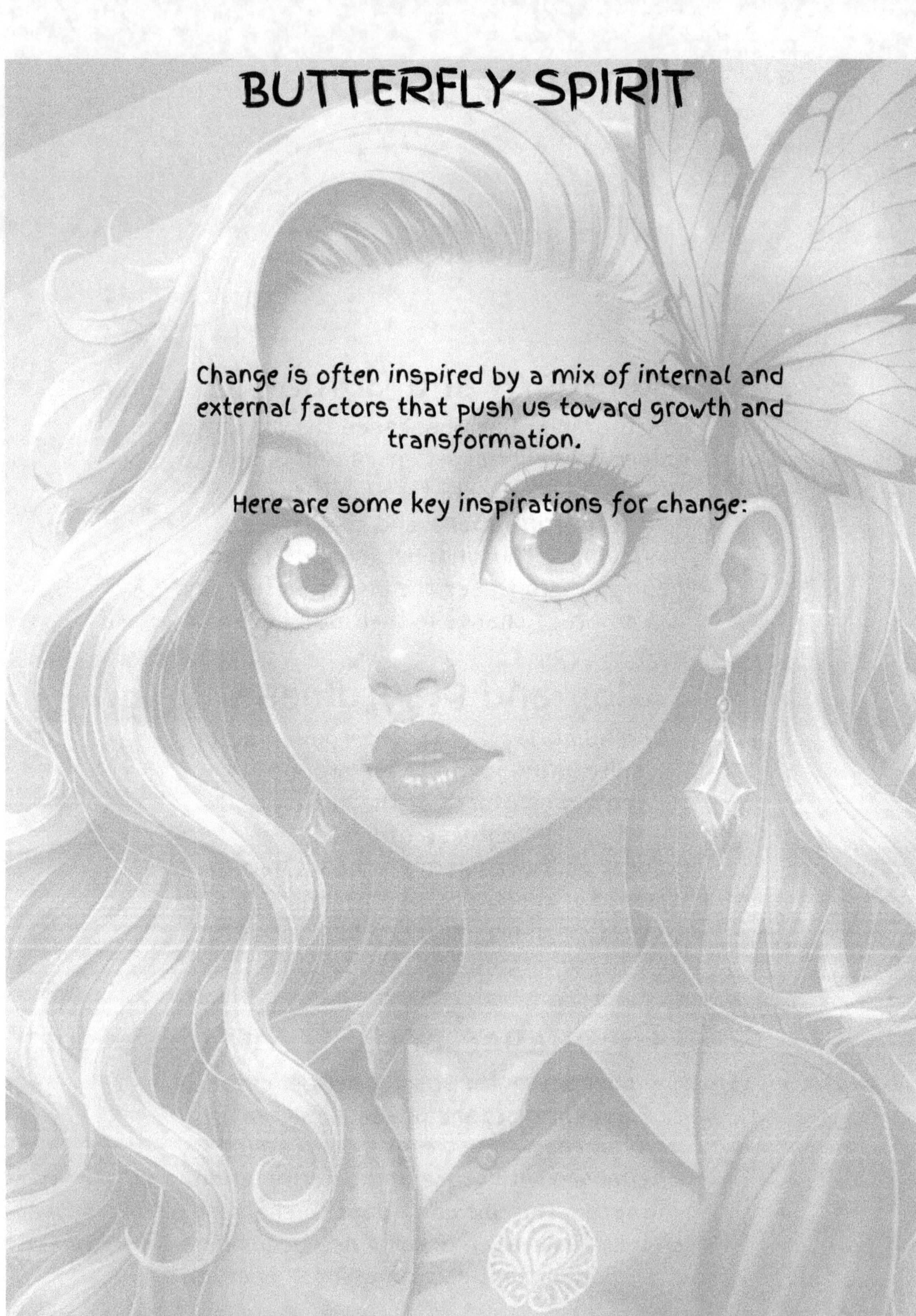

Change is often inspired by a mix of internal and external factors that push us toward growth and transformation.

Here are some key inspirations for change:

BUTTERFLY SPIRIT

New Opportunities:

Encountering new possibilities—like travel, education, or career prospects—can spark change by opening up new horizons and expanding one's perspective.

Self-Reflection:

Time spent reflecting on one's life, values, or goals can lead to realizations that inspire change. This might happen through meditation, journaling, or moments of clarity.

Health and Well-being: Physical and mental health issues, or a desire for better well-being, often push individuals to make lifestyle changes, adopt healthier habits, or find balance.

Curiosity and Adventure:

The human drive to explore new experiences, environments, and ideas can also be a motivator for change. A love for adventure and curiosity often leads to embracing transformation.

Natural Life Cycles: Like the butterfly, people go through natural phases of change due to age, maturity, or shifts in priorities as they navigate different stages of life.

BUTTERFLY SPIRIT

Desire for Growth and Improvement:

Many people change because they feel a deep need to grow, learn, and become better versions of themselves. This could be personal development, career advancement, or spiritual fulfillment.

Life Events:

Significant life events—like a new job, relationship changes, loss, or becoming a parent—can spark a desire to change in response to new roles or realities.

Challenges and Adversity:

Struggles and hardships often force people to adapt. Overcoming adversity often inspires personal transformation, resilience, and the courage to start over.

Inspiration from Others: Seeing others succeed, grow, or change can motivate individuals to seek similar paths. Role models and mentors often inspire change by showcasing what's possible.

Dissatisfaction with the Status Quo:

A sense of dissatisfaction—whether in a job, relationship or with oneself—can ignite the need for change. When people feel stuck or unfulfilled, they often seek new directions.

BUTTERFLY SPIRIT

Butterflies inspire growth through their powerful symbolism of transformation, resilience, and beauty, which resonates deeply with the human experience.

Here are several ways they inspire personal growth:

The butterfly's delicate yet powerful presence reminds us that growth requires change, courage, and trust in the process.

BUTTERFLY SPIRIT

Symbol of Transformation:

The butterfly's *life cycle*—moving from egg to caterpillar, then chrysalis, and finally emerging as a butterfly—mirrors our own capacity for transformation.

It teaches that growth often requires change, even when it's difficult or uncomfortable. Like the butterfly, we must sometimes undergo periods of uncertainty or hardship (the chrysalis stage) before we emerge stronger and more beautiful.

Embracing Change:

Butterflies show that change is a natural part of life and can lead to profound beauty. Their metamorphosis encourages us to embrace transitions rather than fear them, knowing that change is a pathway to becoming the best version of ourselves.

BUTTERFLY SPIRIT

Letting Go of the Old:

A caterpillar must shed its old form to become a butterfly, which reflects the need to let go of outdated mindsets, habits, or limitations. In our own lives, personal growth often requires releasing the past to make room for new opportunities.

Freedom and Expansion:

Once the butterfly emerges, it takes flight with grace and freedom, symbolizing how growth leads to expansion—new perspectives, experiences, and freedom to explore our full potential. This inspires us to spread our wings and embrace life's opportunities without fear.

Beauty in Diversity:

Butterflies come in countless colors and patterns, reminding us that growth doesn't have a single form. Each person's journey is unique, and there is beauty in diversity, both in nature and in personal development.

Living in the Moment:

Butterflies have relatively short lifespans, yet they live fully in each moment. This inspires growth by encouraging us to focus on the present, savor life's beauty, and make the most of every opportunity for learning and development.

BUTTERFLY SPIRIT

Transformation is often triggered by a combination of internal desires and external circumstances. Here are some key factors that can initiate personal transformation:

These triggers often propel individuals into transformative periods, where they evolve in response to new circumstances, challenges, or insights.

BUTTERFLY SPIRIT

Desire for Personal Growth:
A deep longing to improve oneself or to live a more fulfilling life is a powerful trigger for transformation. This can stem from a desire to break free from old habits, reach personal goals, or find purpose and meaning.

Crisis or Adversity:
Challenging situations, such as the loss of a loved one, a health scare, job loss, or emotional trauma, often serve as catalysts for transformation. These experiences force people to re-evaluate their lives, adapt to new realities, and grow stronger as a result.

Discontent with the Status Quo:
Feeling stuck, unfulfilled, or dissatisfied with life can spark a desire for change. Whether it's in a career, relationship, or personal identity, discontent often motivates people to seek new paths and transform their circumstances.

New Experiences or Opportunities:
Major life changes like moving to a new place, starting a new job, or entering a relationship can trigger transformation. These new experiences push individuals out of their comfort zones, offering fresh perspectives and growth opportunities.

Self-Reflection and Awareness:
Moments of deep introspection or life assessment—such as during meditation, journaling, or therapy—often trigger transformation. Gaining insight into one's desires, behaviors, or life patterns helps initiate change from within.

BUTTERFLY SPIRIT

External Influences:

Inspiration from others, whether through mentors, role models, books, or media, can trigger transformation. Witnessing someone else's growth or hearing a profound story can *ignite the belief that change is possible.*

Health or Well-Being Concerns:

Physical or mental health challenges often act as wake-up calls, urging individuals to make significant changes in their lifestyle, mindset, or habits to heal and grow.

Spiritual Awakening:

A spiritual shift or awakening can trigger deep transformation, as individuals seek to align with higher values, purpose, or meaning in life. This can lead to a reassessment of priorities, relationships, and *life choices.*

Milestones or Life Transitions:

Significant life events, such as getting married, having a child, graduating, or turning a certain age, can trigger transformation by shifting priorities and opening new chapters in life.

Sudden Realizations or Epiphanies:

Sometimes transformation is triggered by a sudden moment of clarity—an epiphany or realization about one's life path, relationships, or purpose. These moments can be life-altering, prompting immediate changes.

BUTTERFLY SPIRIT

After growth, several important phases often follow, each building on the progress and transformation achieved.

These stages reflect the ongoing nature of personal development and self-actualization:

Life continues to present challenges, opportunities, and moments for further growth, leading to an ongoing journey of self-improvement.

BUTTERFLY SPIRIT

Reflection and Self-Awareness:

After periods of intense growth, there's often a time of reflection. This involves looking back on how far you've come, appreciating the journey, and becoming more aware of who you are now compared to where you started. This increased self-awareness deepens your connection with your inner self.

Rest and Recovery:

Growth can be challenging and exhausting, so after a significant period of development, it's natural to enter a phase of rest and recovery. This time allows you to recharge and consolidate the changes, giving space to rejuvenate before the next stage of growth begins.

Resilience and Adaptability:

After growth, individuals often become more resilient. With new skills and perspectives, you are better equipped to handle future challenges. Growth strengthens your adaptability, enabling you to face life's ups and downs with greater ease.

Continuous Evolution:

Growth is not a linear process—it's cyclical. After one phase of growth, there is always the potential for new transformations. Life continues to present challenges, opportunities, and moments for further growth, leading to an ongoing journey of self-improvement.

BUTTERFLY SPIRIT

Maturity and Stability:

After growth, a sense of maturity often emerges. This involves integrating lessons learned, finding balance, and achieving a stable foundation. It's a period of deeper understanding and emotional stability, where you apply the wisdom gained through growth.

Mastery:

Growth leads to mastering new skills, mindsets, or life challenges. This stage is marked by confidence and competence in areas where you once struggled. Mastery doesn't mean the journey is over, but it signifies that you've gained control and proficiency.

Contentment and Fulfillment:

With growth comes a sense of fulfillment and satisfaction. Having worked through challenges or personal changes, you may feel more aligned with your values, purpose, and goals. This leads to a deeper sense of contentment in life.

Contribution and Sharing:

Once personal growth is achieved, many people feel compelled to share their knowledge or help others. This stage is about giving back—mentoring, teaching, or supporting others in their own journeys of growth. It reflects a desire to make a positive impact on the world around you.

New Goals and Aspirations:

Growth often leads to new perspectives and opens up new possibilities. After achieving one stage of growth, you may find yourself setting fresh goals, exploring new interests, or pursuing different aspirations. The cycle of growth continues as you evolve in new directions.

BUTTERFLY SPIRIT

Building Relationships
Nurturing Connections: She forms new, supportive relationships that inspire her growth and provide encouragement. Surrounding herself with like-minded individuals fosters a sense of community and belonging.

Sharing Wisdom:
As she transforms, she shares her insights and experiences with others, becoming a mentor and guiding light for those on similar journeys.

Integration of Changes
Self-Reflection: Regularly reflecting on her journey helps her recognize how far she's come, integrating the lessons learned into her life.

Living Authentically:
Embracing her true self allows her to live authentically, embodying the qualities she has cultivated throughout her transformation.

Symbolic Metamorphosis
Physical Representation: In moments of deep transformation, she might experience a symbolic metamorphosis, feeling lighter and more radiant, much like a butterfly emerging from a chrysalis.

Manifesting Powers:
As she transforms, her butterfly spirit powers may become more pronounced, allowing her to help others on their journeys of growth.

BUTTERFLY SPIRIT

Through these steps, she undergoes a beautiful and profound transformation, continually evolving into the best version of herself.

This process reflects the essence of a butterfly's metamorphosis, showcasing resilience, adaptability, and the power of embracing change.

As a human butterfly spirit, she uses her unique powers to vanquish challengers by embodying resilience, wisdom, and transformation.

Here's how she harnesses her abilities in the face of adversity:

BUTTERFLY SPIRIT

Empathetic Understanding

Gaining Insight: She employs her deep empathy to understand the motivations and fears of her challengers. By knowing their weaknesses, she can respond strategically and compassionately, often diffusing conflicts before they escalate.

Transforming Enmity:

Rather than confronting challengers with aggression, she seeks common ground and attempts to transform adversarial relationships into alliances through understanding and communication.

Resilience and Adaptability

Bouncing Back: When faced with challenges, she draws upon her resilience to bounce back from setbacks. Her ability to adapt to changing circumstances allows her to remain flexible and resourceful in finding solutions.

Overcoming Obstacles:

She embraces challenges as opportunities for growth, using her experiences to fuel her determination and strength. This inner fortitude intimidates her challengers, as they realize she cannot be easily defeated.

BUTTERFLY SPIRIT

Through these methods, the human butterfly spirit not only vanquishes her challengers but also transforms conflicts into opportunities for growth and connection.

Her powers reflect the essence of transformation and resilience, allowing her to navigate challenges with grace and strength.

BUTTERFLY SPIRIT

What are Nature Prayers?

Nature prayers are prayers or spiritual practices that connect a person with the natural world.
These prayers often express gratitude, reverence, and respect for the elements of nature—such as the earth, water, sky, plants, animals, and the cycles of life.

They recognize the beauty and power of nature as a reflection of the divine and can involve requests for guidance, healing, protection, or wisdom from nature's forces.

Nature prayers can take many forms, including:

Gratitude prayers for the beauty and sustenance provided by nature (like food, water, and air).
Blessings over plants, animals, or landscapes.

Meditations or moments of silence in natural settings, focusing on the elements like wind, rain, or sunlight.

Rituals performed during specific natural events like the solstice, equinox, or phases of the moon.

BUTTERFLY SPIRIT

People who practice nature prayers often *feel* a deeper connection to the earth and see it as a *living*, spiritual entity that deserves care and respect.

In some traditions, nature prayers are linked to animism, indigenous spirituality, or pagan practices, while in others, they are seen as an extension of one's relationship with God or the divine, manifesting through the natural world.

BUTTERFLY SPIRIT

Why Are Nature Prayers Important?

Connection to the Earth: Nature prayers help people reconnect with the earth and its rhythms. In today's fast-paced world, we can easily become disconnected from the environment. Praying through or to nature reminds us that we are part of a larger ecosystem and helps foster a sense of unity with all living things.

Gratitude and Reverence:

These prayers promote gratitude for the resources we receive from nature—food, water, shelter, and the air we breathe. Practicing gratitude can lead to a more mindful and appreciative way of living, encouraging us to care for the earth and its inhabitants.

Healing and Grounding:

Nature has long been associated with healing. By focusing prayers on the natural elements—like asking for the calming energy of the wind or the healing power of water—people often feel more grounded, balanced, and at peace.

Nature prayers can be used to restore emotional, physical, or spiritual health.

BUTTERFLY SPIRIT

In essence, nature prayers are important because they offer a way to harmonize with the earth and its sacredness, fostering a deeper understanding of our role in the world and our connection to both the natural and spiritual realms.

BUTTERFLY SPIRIT

Butterfly Spirit-Inspired Nature Praying
Rituals
These rituals align with the transformative,
beautiful, and ambitious energy of Butterfly
Spirit. Each ritual centers on connecting with
nature, embracing change, and drawing
strength from the cycles of life, just like the
butterfly.

BUTTERFLY SPIRIT

THE CHRYSALIS RENEWAL RITUAL

(For Personal Transformation)

This ritual is designed to help you embrace transformation in your life, just like a butterfly shedding its old form to reveal a new one.

It can be performed when you feel stuck or in need of change.

Materials:

A quiet, outdoor space
A soft blanket or cushion
A small mirror
A candle (preferably white or blue)
Flowers (any type that feels meaningful to you)

BUTTERFLY SPIRIT

THE CHRYSALIS RENEWAL RITUAL

Steps:
Find a Space in Nature: Choose a space where you feel calm, surrounded by trees, flowers, or open skies.

Prepare Your Circle:
Lay down the blanket, placing the flowers around you in a circle. Place the mirror in front of you, symbolizing self-reflection, and light the candle, representing the light of transformation.

Grounding:
Close your eyes, breathe deeply, and imagine roots growing from your feet into the earth. Let yourself feel grounded, and supported by the earth's energy.

Recite the Prayer:
"Butterfly Spirit, guide me through this time of transformation.

As the earth changes with the seasons,
As the butterfly emerges from the chrysalis,
Let me shed the old and embrace my new form.
I trust in the process of growth, and I welcome the beauty of my rebirth.

Just as the wind carries the butterfly, may your grace carry me to my highest self."
Mirror Reflection: Gaze into the mirror, reflecting on who you are and who you wish to become. Speak aloud about the qualities you want to embody.

Release and Accept:
Blow out the candle, symbolizing the end of your old self. Stand up, raise your arms to the sky, and feel the energy of the transformation pouring into you. Visualize yourself as a butterfly, free and beautiful.

BUTTERFLY SPIRIT

The Flight of Ambition Ritual

(For Achieving Goals)

This ritual is for when you need a boost of energy and focus to achieve your ambitions.

It connects the power of nature with the determination of Butterfly Spirit.

Materials:
Feathers (to symbolize wings)
A clear quartz crystal (for clarity and focus)
A journal and pen
A small bowl of water

A natural space with open air, such as a meadow or hilltop

BUTTERFLY SPIRIT

The Flight of Ambition Ritual

(For Achieving Goals)

Steps:
Create an Altar:
Set up your altar on the ground, placing the feathers, crystal, and bowl of water in front of you.

Grounding and Breathing:
Sit on the ground, close your eyes, and take deep breaths. Imagine the wind moving around you, like wings fluttering.

Prayer of Ambition:
"Butterfly Spirit, who rises with grace and power,
Grant me the strength to soar toward my goals.
As you break free from limitation, so too shall I break through my fears.
I call upon the wind to carry me forward,
And the earth to give me strength in my pursuit.
With clear vision, I will achieve all that I desire."

Visualization:
Hold the crystal in your hand and close your eyes. Visualize your goal clearly in your mind. Imagine yourself already achieving it, feeling the excitement of success.

Feather Offering:
Lay the feathers on the ground as an offering to Butterfly Spirit, asking for her guidance in helping you take flight in your ambitions.

Water Reflection:
Dip your fingers in the bowl of water, sprinkling it on the earth around you, symbolizing the nurturing of your dreams.

BUTTERFLY SPIRIT

THE GARDEN OF KINDNESS RITUAL

(For Healing Relationships)

This ritual helps cultivate kindness and healing
in your relationships, drawing from Butterfly
Spirit's compassion and grace.

Materials:

Seeds (any type of flower or plant that speaks
to you)
A small patch of soil
A blue or green cloth
A bowl of water

BUTTERFLY SPIRIT

THE GARDEN OF KINDNESS RITUAL

Steps:

Prepare the Space:
Lay the blue or green cloth on the ground and place the seeds and bowl of water on it. Choose a patch of soil where you can plant the seeds.
1. Planting the Seeds: Hold the seeds in your hand and speak softly to them, expressing your hopes for healing and kindness in your relationships.

Prayer for Healing:
"Butterfly Spirit, you who dances upon the wind,
Teach me the art of grace and gentleness.
As I plant these seeds, may love and understanding grow.
May the winds of forgiveness blow between me and others,
May the waters of kindness flow freely in our hearts.
I call on your healing wings to mend what is broken,
And to lift our spirits with compassion."
Plant the Seeds: Place the seeds into the soil, one by one, imagining each seed as a moment of kindness or understanding between you and someone else.

Watering:
Pour the water over the seeds, symbolizing the nurturing and growth of love and forgiveness. Whisper words of peace as you do this, sending healing energy to all your relationships.

Closing:
Fold the cloth and keep it as a reminder to tend to your relationships with care, just as you tend to the seeds you've planted.

BUTTERFLY SPIRIT

THE MOONLIT EMERGENCE RITUAL

(For Embracing Your True Self)

This ritual taps into the phases of the moon, representing the cycles of growth and emergence, just like Butterfly Spirit's transformation from caterpillar to butterfly.

Materials:

A moonstone or any reflective stone
A silver or white candle
A journal and pen
A quiet, outdoor space under the moonlight

BUTTERFLY SPIRIT

THE MOONLIT EMERGENCE RITUAL

(For Embracing Your True Self)
Steps:
Prepare for the Moon's Energy:

Choose a night when the moon is visible. Set up your space outdoors, lighting a silver or white candle.

Reflection Under the Moon:

Hold the moonstone in your hands and look up at the moon, letting its light wash over you. Close your eyes and imagine the moon reflecting your true self—your potential, your beauty, your strength.

Prayer for Emergence: "Butterfly Spirit, illuminated by the moon's light,
Help me to shed my false layers and emerge as my true self.
Just as you transform in the stillness,
So too do I bloom under the moon's glow.
Guide me through the shadows,
And reveal the beauty that lies within.
With every phase, I will rise closer to my true form."
Writing Your Emergence: In your journal, write down who you truly are and what you wish to reveal to the world. Allow the moonlight to inspire you, helping you recognize your hidden beauty.

Closing:

Blow out the candle and hold the moonstone to your heart, affirming that you are constantly growing and evolving into your best self.

BUTTERFLY SPIRIT

These rituals honor the energy of
Butterfly Spirit and the natural
world, fostering growth, ambition,
healing, and self-awareness.

Through them, you connect with
the cycles of nature and your own
inner strength, just as Butterfly
Spirit does in her journey of
transformation.

BUTTERFLY SPIRIT

✹ Nature Connection Prayer Page ✹

Date: ____________________________

🌀 Nature Prayers for Transformation:
Write your own nature-inspired prayer for growth and abundance:

☑ Check off when practiced in nature:
Meditated in a natural setting.
Said my prayer outdoors.
Observed nature's beauty and abundance.

BUTTERFLY SPIRIT

Celebrating Small Wins Page

Date: ________________________

🔺 Today's Achievements:
List your wins, big or small:

🌈 Celebration Actions:

What will I do to celebrate my progress?

Empowering Affirmations:
Create affirmations to replace limiting beliefs:
I am worthy of abundance.

BUTTERFLY SPIRIT

🌀 Abundance Mindset Reflections 🌀
Date: _______________________________
🌷 Limiting Beliefs to Release:
What beliefs do I want to let go of?

🖤 Gratitude Checklist 🖤
Date: _______________________________
🌼 Today, I am grateful for:
List five things you appreciate today.

⚓ Gratitude Actions:
Check all that apply today!
I expressed gratitude to someone.
I wrote in my gratitude journal.
I shared my appreciation on social media.
I did something kind for myself.
I acknowledged a personal achievement.

BUTTERFLY SPIRIT

❀ Transformation Goals Page ❀
Date: _______________________________
My Transformation Intentions:
What changes do I want to embrace?

Visualizing My Abundance:
Picture what success looks like for you:

BUTTERFLY SPIRIT

🦋 Inspired Action Checklist 🦋

Date: _______________________

🦋 Actions to Attract Abundance:
What steps will I take today?

🦋 Networking Opportunities:
Individuals to connect with:

✓ Check off actions taken:

☐ Reached out to someone.

☐ Attended a networking event.

☐ Engaged in a community project.

BUTTERFLY SPIRIT

Here's a refined set of *fill-in-the-blank*, checklist grid journal pages that emphasize beauty and detail, incorporating the butterfly spirit theme.

These pages are designed to be functional yet visually appealing, encouraging a joyful journaling experience.

Butterfly Spirit Journal Pages
🦋 Transformation Goals Page 🦋
Date: _______________________
My Transformation Intentions:
What changes do I want to embrace?

Visualizing My Abundance:
Picture what success looks like for you:

💚 Gratitude Checklist 💚

Date: _______________________
Today, I am grateful for:
List five things you appreciate today.

🦋 Gratitude Actions:
Check all that apply today!
I expressed gratitude to someone.
I wrote in my gratitude journal.
I shared my appreciation on social media.
I did something kind for myself.
I acknowledged a personal achievement.

BUTTERFLY SPIRIT

Weekly Manifestation Script
Preparation
Find a quiet space and take a few deep breaths to center yourself.
1. Opening Invocation
"Dear Universe, I open my heart and mind to receive the blessings of my desires. I trust in the process of manifestation."
2. Reflection on Desires
This week, I desire:

____
____
____

3. Visualization
(Close your eyes and visualize your desires as already achieved.)
Feel the joy and gratitude as if they are yours now.
4. Affirmations
"I am worthy of my desires."
"Abundance flows to me effortlessly."
"I trust the timing of my manifestations."
5. Gratitude
"Thank you, Universe, for all my blessings and for the desires that are on their way to me."
6. Action Steps
This week, I will:

____
____
____

7. Closing Intention
"I trust that my desires are manifesting in perfect timing. So it is, and so it shall be."

BUTTERFLY SPIRIT

Weekly Manifestation Ritual Script
Preparation
Find a quiet space where you can sit comfortably without distractions.
Gather items that resonate with you (e.g., crystals, candles, or meaningful objects).
Take a few deep breaths to center yourself.
1. Opening Invocation
(Speak or write this aloud)
"Dear Universe, God, and my higher self, I come to you with an open heart and mind. I acknowledge the power of my intentions and the beauty of my desires. I am grateful for this moment to align with my true self and manifest my dreams."
2. Reflection on Desires
(Take a moment to reflect on the following questions. You can write your responses in a journal.)
What are my desires this week?

Why are these desires important to me?

BUTTERFLY SPIRIT

3. Visualization
(Close your eyes and visualize your desires as if they have already manifested.)
Imagine how it feels to achieve each desire.
Engage all your senses—what do you see, hear, feel, and smell?
Spend 5-10 minutes in this visualization, allowing the feelings of joy and fulfillment to wash over you.
4. Affirmations
(Repeat the following affirmations, either aloud or silently, believing in their truth.)
"I am worthy of all my desires and dreams."
"Abundance flows to me effortlessly and easily."
"I trust the process of manifestation, and I am open to receiving."
"I am a magnet for love, success, and prosperity."
5. Gratitude Practice
(Take a moment to express gratitude for what you already have and for what is coming.)
"Thank you, Universe, for the blessings in my life."
"I am grateful for the opportunities that align with my desires."
"Thank you for supporting me on this journey of manifestation."
6. Action Steps
(Identify actionable steps you can take this week to support your manifestation.)
What will I do this week to move closer to my desires?

BUTTERFLY SPIRIT

CHECK OUT ALL MY BOOKS!

BUTTERFLY SPIRIT

❧ Nature Connection Prayer Page ❧

Date: _______________________________

🖋 Nature Prayers for Transformation:
Write your own nature-inspired prayer for growth and abundance:

☑ Check off when practiced in nature:
Meditated in a natural setting.
Said my prayer outdoors.
Observed nature's beauty and abundance.

BUTTERFLY SPIRIT

Celebrating Small Wins Page

Date: ____________________________

☙ Today's Achievements:
List your wins, big or small:

⟆ Celebration Actions:

What will I do to celebrate my progress?

Empowering Affirmations:
Create affirmations to replace limiting beliefs:
I am worthy of abundance.

BUTTERFLY SPIRIT

🌈 Abundance Mindset Reflections 🌈
Date: _______________________________
🪷 Limiting Beliefs to Release:
What beliefs do I want to let go of?

💜 Gratitude Checklist 💜
Date: _______________________________
☀ Today, I am grateful for:
List five things you appreciate today.

Gratitude Actions:
Check all that apply today!
I expressed gratitude to someone.
I wrote in my gratitude journal.
I shared my appreciation on social media.
I did something kind for myself.
I acknowledged a personal achievement.

BUTTERFLY SPIRIT

❃ Transformation Goals Page ❃
Date: _______________________________
My Transformation Intentions:
What changes do I want to embrace?

Visualizing My Abundance:
Picture what success looks like for you:

BUTTERFLY SPIRIT

🦋 Inspired Action Checklist 🦋

Date: _______________________________

Actions to Attract Abundance:
What steps will I take today?

Networking Opportunities:
Individuals to connect with:

✓ Check off actions taken:

☐ Reached out to someone.

☐ Attended a networking event.

☐ Engaged in a community project.

BUTTERFLY SPIRIT

Here's a refined set of fill-in-the-blank, checklist grid journal pages that emphasize beauty and detail, incorporating the butterfly spirit theme.

These pages are designed to be functional yet visually appealing, encouraging a joyful journaling experience.

Butterfly Spirit Journal Pages
🦋 Transformation Goals Page 🦋
Date: _______________________
My Transformation Intentions:
What changes do I want to embrace?

Visualizing My Abundance:
Picture what success looks like for you:

💜 Gratitude Checklist 💜

Date: _______________________
Today, I am grateful for:
List five things you appreciate today.

Gratitude Actions:
Check all that apply today!
I expressed gratitude to someone.
I wrote in my gratitude journal.
I shared my appreciation on social media.
I did something kind for myself.
I acknowledged a personal achievement.

BUTTERFLY SPIRIT

Weekly Manifestation Script
Preparation
Find a quiet space and take a few deep breaths to center yourself.
1. Opening Invocation
"Dear Universe, I open my heart and mind to receive the blessings of my
desires. I trust in the process of manifestation."
2. Reflection on Desires
This week, I desire:

----

3. Visualization
(Close your eyes and visualize your desires as already achieved.)
Feel the joy and gratitude as if they are yours now.
4. Affirmations
"I am worthy of my desires."
"Abundance flows to me effortlessly."
"I trust the timing of my manifestations."
5. Gratitude
"Thank you, Universe, for all my blessings and for the desires that are on
their way to me."
6. Action Steps
This week, I will:

----

7. Closing Intention
"I trust that my desires are manifesting in perfect timing. So it is, and so it
shall be."

BUTTERFLY SPIRIT

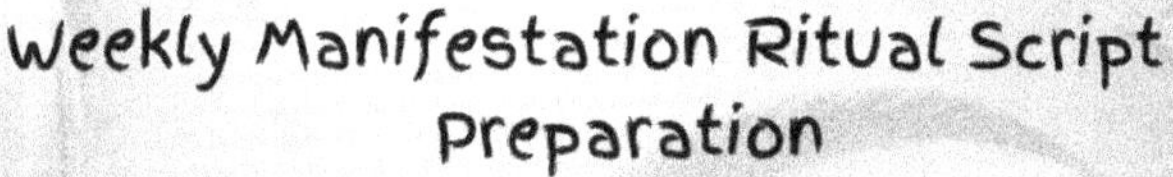

Weekly Manifestation Ritual Script
Preparation
Find a quiet space where you can sit comfortably without distractions.
Gather items that resonate with you (e.g., crystals, candles, or meaningful objects).
Take a few deep breaths to center yourself.
1. Opening Invocation
(Speak or write this aloud)
"Dear Universe, God, and my higher self, I come to you with an open heart and mind. I acknowledge the power of my intentions and the beauty of my desires. I am grateful for this moment to align with my true self and manifest my dreams."
2. Reflection on Desires
(Take a moment to reflect on the following questions. You can write your responses in a journal.)
What are my desires this week?

Why are these desires important to me?

BUTTERFLY SPIRIT

3. Visualization
(Close your eyes and visualize your desires as if they have already manifested.)
Imagine how it feels to achieve each desire.
Engage all your senses—what do you see, hear, feel, and smell?
Spend 5-10 minutes in this visualization, allowing the feelings of joy and fulfillment to wash over you.

4. Affirmations
(Repeat the following affirmations, either aloud or silently, believing in their truth.)
"I am worthy of all my desires and dreams."
"Abundance flows to me effortlessly and easily."
"I trust the process of manifestation, and I am open to receiving."
"I am a magnet for love, success, and prosperity."

5. Gratitude Practice
(Take a moment to express gratitude for what you already have and for what is coming.)
"Thank you, Universe, for the blessings in my life."
"I am grateful for the opportunities that align with my desires."
"Thank you for supporting me on this journey of manifestation."

6. Action Steps
(Identify actionable steps you can take this week to support your manifestation.)
What will I do this week to move closer to my desires?

BUTTERFLY SPIRIT
CHECK OUT ALL MY BOOKS!

BUTTERFLY SPIRIT

✿ Nature Connection Prayer Page ✿

Date: _______________________

🐚 Nature Prayers for Transformation:

Write your own nature-inspired prayer for growth and abundance:

☑ Check off when practiced in nature:

Meditated in a natural setting.

Said my prayer outdoors.

Observed nature's beauty and abundance.

BUTTERFLY SPIRIT

Celebrating Small Wins Page

Date: ____________________

Today's Achievements:
List your wins, big or small:

Celebration Actions:

What will I do to celebrate my progress?

Empowering Affirmations:
Create affirmations to replace limiting beliefs:
I am worthy of abundance.

BUTTERFLY SPIRIT

🌀 Abundance Mindset Reflections 🌀
Date: _______________________________
❀ Limiting Beliefs to Release:
What beliefs do I want to let go of?

💗 Gratitude Checklist 💗
Date: _______________________________
❀ Today, I am grateful for:
List five things you appreciate today.

⚓ Gratitude Actions:
Check all that apply today!
I expressed gratitude to someone.
I wrote in my gratitude journal.
I shared my appreciation on social media.
I did something kind for myself.
I acknowledged a personal achievement.

BUTTERFLY SPIRIT

🦋 Transformation Goals Page 🦋
Date: _______________________________
My Transformation Intentions:
What changes do I want to embrace?

____
____
____

Visualizing My Abundance:
Picture what success looks like for you:

____
____

BUTTERFLY SPIRIT

🦋 Inspired Action Checklist 🦋
Date: _______________________
Actions to Attract Abundance:
What steps will I take today?

Networking Opportunities:
Individuals to connect with:

✓ Check off actions taken:

☐ Reached out to someone.

☐ Attended a networking event.

☐ Engaged in a community project.

BUTTERFLY SPIRIT

Here's a refined set of fill-in-the-blank, checklist grid journal pages that emphasize beauty and detail, incorporating the butterfly spirit theme.

These pages are designed to be functional yet visually appealing, encouraging a joyful journaling experience.

Butterfly Spirit Journal Pages
🦋 Transformation Goals Page 🦋
Date: ______________________________
My Transformation Intentions:
What changes do I want to embrace?

Visualizing My Abundance:
Picture what success looks like for you:

🖤 Gratitude Checklist 🖤

Date: ______________________________
Today, I am grateful for:
List five things you appreciate today.

Gratitude Actions:
Check all that apply today!
I expressed gratitude to someone.
I wrote in my gratitude journal.
I shared my appreciation on social media.
I did something kind for myself.
I acknowledged a personal achievement.

BUTTERFLY SPIRIT

Weekly Manifestation Script
Preparation
Find a quiet space and take a few deep breaths to center yourself.
1. Opening Invocation
"Dear Universe, I open my heart and mind to receive the blessings of my desires. I trust in the process of manifestation."
2. Reflection on Desires
This week, I desire:

____
____
____

3. Visualization
(Close your eyes and visualize your desires as already achieved.)
Feel the joy and gratitude as if they are yours now.
4. Affirmations
"I am worthy of my desires."
"Abundance flows to me effortlessly."
"I trust the timing of my manifestations."
5. Gratitude
"Thank you, Universe, for all my blessings and for the desires that are on their way to me."
6. Action Steps
This week, I will:

____
____
____

7. Closing Intention
"I trust that my desires are manifesting in perfect timing. So it is, and so it shall be."

BUTTERFLY SPIRIT

Weekly Manifestation Ritual Script
Preparation
Find a quiet space where you can sit comfortably without distractions.
Gather items that resonate with you (e.g., crystals, candles, or meaningful objects).
Take a few deep breaths to center yourself.
1. Opening Invocation
(Speak or write this aloud)
"Dear Universe, God, and my higher self, I come to you with an open heart and mind. I acknowledge the power of my intentions and the beauty of my desires. I am grateful for this moment to align with my true self and manifest my dreams."
2. Reflection on Desires
(Take a moment to reflect on the following questions. You can write your responses in a journal.)
What are my desires this week?

Why are these desires important to me?

BUTTERFLY SPIRIT

3. Visualization
(Close your eyes and visualize your desires as if they have already manifested.)
Imagine how it feels to achieve each desire.
Engage all your senses—what do you see, hear, feel, and smell?
Spend 5-10 minutes in this visualization, allowing the feelings of joy and fulfillment to wash over you.

4. Affirmations
(Repeat the following affirmations, either aloud or silently, believing in their truth.)
"I am worthy of all my desires and dreams."
"Abundance flows to me effortlessly and easily."
"I trust the process of manifestation, and I am open to receiving."
"I am a magnet for love, success, and prosperity."

5. Gratitude Practice
(Take a moment to express gratitude for what you already have and for what is coming.)
"Thank you, Universe, for the blessings in my life."
"I am grateful for the opportunities that align with my desires."
"Thank you for supporting me on this journey of manifestation."

6. Action Steps
(Identify actionable steps you can take this week to support your manifestation.)
What will I do this week to move closer to my desires?

BUTTERFLY SPIRIT
CHECK OUT ALL MY BOOKS!

BUTTERFLY SPIRIT

🌿 Nature Connection Prayer Page 🌿

Date: ______________________________

Nature Prayers for Transformation:

Write your own nature-inspired prayer for growth and abundance:

____

____

☑ Check off when practiced in nature:

Meditated in a natural setting.

Said my prayer outdoors.

Observed nature's beauty and abundance.

BUTTERFLY SPIRIT

Celebrating Small Wins Page

Date: ____________________________

Today's Achievements:
List your wins, big or small:

____

____

____

Celebration Actions:

What will I do to celebrate my progress?

____

____

Empowering Affirmations:
Create affirmations to replace limiting beliefs:
I am worthy of abundance.

____

____

BUTTERFLY SPIRIT

🌈 Abundance Mindset Reflections 🌈
Date: ______________________________
🌱 Limiting Beliefs to Release:
What beliefs do I want to let go of?

💜 Gratitude Checklist 💜
Date: ____________________________
🌼 Today, I am grateful for:
List five things you appreciate today.

Gratitude Actions:
Check all that apply today!
I expressed gratitude to someone.
I wrote in my gratitude journal.
I shared my appreciation on social media.
I did something kind for myself.
I acknowledged a personal achievement.

BUTTERFLY SPIRIT

🦋 Transformation Goals Page 🦋
Date: _______________________________
My Transformation Intentions:
What changes do I want to embrace?

Visualizing My Abundance:
Picture what success looks like for you:

BUTTERFLY SPIRIT

🦋 Inspired Action Checklist 🦋

Date: _______________________________

Actions to Attract Abundance:
What steps will I take today?

Networking Opportunities:
Individuals to connect with:

☑ Check off actions taken:

☐ Reached out to someone.

☐ Attended a networking event.

☐ Engaged in a community project.

BUTTERFLY SPIRIT

Here's a refined set of fill-in-the-blank, checklist grid journal pages that emphasize beauty and detail, incorporating the butterfly spirit theme.

These pages are designed to be functional yet visually appealing, encouraging a joyful journaling experience.

Butterfly Spirit Journal Pages
✖ Transformation Goals Page ✖
Date: _______________________
My Transformation Intentions:
What changes do I want to embrace?

____
____
____

Visualizing My Abundance:
Picture what success looks like for you:

____
____

🖤 Gratitude Checklist 🖤

Date: _______________________
Today, I am grateful for:
List five things you appreciate today.

____
____
____
____
____

Gratitude Actions:
Check all that apply today!
I expressed gratitude to someone.
I wrote in my gratitude journal.
I shared my appreciation on social media.
I did something kind for myself.
I acknowledged a personal achievement.

BUTTERFLY SPIRIT

Weekly Manifestation Script
Preparation
Find a quiet space and take a few deep breaths to center yourself.
1. Opening Invocation
"Dear Universe, I open my heart and mind to receive the blessings of my desires. I trust in the process of manifestation."
2. Reflection on Desires
This week, I desire:

----

3. Visualization
(Close your eyes and visualize your desires as already achieved.)
Feel the joy and gratitude as if they are yours now.
4. Affirmations
"I am worthy of my desires."
"Abundance flows to me effortlessly."
"I trust the timing of my manifestations."
5. Gratitude
"Thank you, Universe, for all my blessings and for the desires that are on their way to me."
6. Action Steps
This week, I will:

----

7. Closing Intention
"I trust that my desires are manifesting in perfect timing. So it is, and so it shall be."

BUTTERFLY SPIRIT

Weekly Manifestation Ritual Script
Preparation
Find a quiet space where you can sit comfortably without distractions.
Gather items that resonate with you (e.g., crystals, candles, or meaningful objects).
Take a few deep breaths to center yourself.
1. Opening Invocation
(Speak or write this aloud)
"Dear Universe, God, and my higher self, I come to you with an open heart and mind. I acknowledge the power of my intentions and the beauty of my desires. I am grateful for this moment to align with my true self and manifest my dreams."
2. Reflection on Desires
(Take a moment to reflect on the following questions. You can write your responses in a journal.)
What are my desires this week?

Why are these desires important to me?

BUTTERFLY SPIRIT

3. Visualization
(Close your eyes and visualize your desires as if they have already
manifested.)
Imagine how it feels to achieve each desire.
Engage all your senses—what do you see, hear, feel, and smell?
Spend 5-10 minutes in this visualization, allowing the feelings of joy and
fulfillment to wash over you.

4. Affirmations
(Repeat the following affirmations, either aloud or silently, believing in their
truth.)
"I am worthy of all my desires and dreams."
"Abundance flows to me effortlessly and easily."
"I trust the process of manifestation, and I am open to receiving."
"I am a magnet for love, success, and prosperity."

5. Gratitude Practice
(Take a moment to express gratitude for what you already have and for
what is coming.)
"Thank you, Universe, for the blessings in my life."
"I am grateful for the opportunities that align with my desires."
"Thank you for supporting me on this journey of manifestation."

6. Action Steps
(Identify actionable steps you can take this week to support your
manifestation.)
What will I do this week to move closer to my desires?

BUTTERFLY SPIRIT
CHECK OUT ALL MY BOOKS!

BUTTERFLY SPIRIT

❧ Nature Connection Prayer Page ❧

Date: ______________________________

❧ Nature Prayers for Transformation:
Write your own nature-inspired prayer for growth and abundance:

☑ Check off when practiced in nature:
Meditated in a natural setting.
Said my prayer outdoors.
Observed nature's beauty and abundance.

BUTTERFLY SPIRIT

Celebrating Small Wins Page
Date: ______________________________
Today's Achievements:
List your wins, big or small:

____
____
____

Celebration Actions:
What will I do to celebrate my progress?

____
____

Empowering Affirmations:
Create affirmations to replace limiting beliefs:
I am worthy of abundance.

____
____

BUTTERFLY SPIRIT

🌈 Abundance Mindset Reflections 🌈
Date: ______________________________
🧘 Limiting Beliefs to Release:
What beliefs do I want to let go of?

💜 Gratitude Checklist 💜
Date: ______________________________
🌼 Today, I am grateful for:
List five things you appreciate today.

🕯 Gratitude Actions:
Check all that apply today!
I expressed gratitude to someone.
I wrote in my gratitude journal.
I shared my appreciation on social media.
I did something kind for myself.
I acknowledged a personal achievement.

BUTTERFLY SPIRIT

🦋 Transformation Goals Page 🦋

Date: _______________________________

My Transformation Intentions:
What changes do I want to embrace?

Visualizing My Abundance:
Picture what success looks like for you:

BUTTERFLY SPIRIT

🦋 Inspired Action Checklist 🦋

Date: _______________________________

🦋 Actions to Attract Abundance:
What steps will I take today?

🦋 Networking Opportunities:
Individuals to connect with:

✓ Check off actions taken:

☐ Reached out to someone.

☐ Attended a networking event.

☐ Engaged in a community project.

BUTTERFLY SPIRIT

Here's a refined set of *fill-in-the-blank*, checklist grid journal pages that emphasize beauty and detail, incorporating the butterfly spirit theme.

These pages are designed to be functional yet visually appealing, encouraging a joyful journaling experience.

Butterfly Spirit Journal Pages
🦋 Transformation Goals Page 🦋
Date: _______________________
My Transformation Intentions:
What changes do I want to embrace?

____
____
____

Visualizing My Abundance:
Picture what success looks like for you:

____
____

🖤 Gratitude Checklist 🖤

Date: _______________________
Today, I am grateful for:
List five things you appreciate today.

____
____
____
____
____

Gratitude Actions:
Check all that apply today!
I expressed gratitude to someone.
I wrote in my gratitude journal.
I shared my appreciation on social media.
I did something kind for myself.
I acknowledged a personal achievement.

BUTTERFLY SPIRIT

Weekly Manifestation Script
Preparation
Find a quiet space and take a few deep breaths to center yourself.
1. Opening Invocation
"Dear Universe, I open my heart and mind to receive the blessings of my desires. I trust in the process of manifestation."
2. Reflection on Desires
This week, I desire:

____

____

____

3. Visualization
(Close your eyes and visualize your desires as already achieved.)
Feel the joy and gratitude as if they are yours now.
4. Affirmations
"I am worthy of my desires."
"Abundance flows to me effortlessly."
"I trust the timing of my manifestations."
5. Gratitude
"Thank you, Universe, for all my blessings and for the desires that are on their way to me."
6. Action Steps
This week, I will:

____

____

____

7. Closing Intention
"I trust that my desires are manifesting in perfect timing. So it is, and so it shall be."

BUTTERFLY SPIRIT

Weekly Manifestation Ritual Script
Preparation
Find a quiet space where you can sit comfortably without distractions.
Gather items that resonate with you (e.g., crystals, candles, or meaningful objects).
Take a few deep breaths to center yourself.
1. Opening Invocation
(Speak or write this aloud)
"Dear Universe, God, and my higher self, I come to you with an open heart and mind. I acknowledge the power of my intentions and the beauty of my desires. I am grateful for this moment to align with my true self and manifest my dreams."
2. Reflection on Desires
(Take a moment to reflect on the following questions. You can write your responses in a journal.)
What are my desires this week?

Why are these desires important to me?

BUTTERFLY SPIRIT

3. Visualization
(Close your eyes and visualize your desires as if they have already manifested.)
Imagine how it feels to achieve each desire.
Engage all your senses—what do you see, hear, feel, and smell?
Spend 5-10 minutes in this visualization, allowing the feelings of joy and fulfillment to wash over you.

4. Affirmations
(Repeat the following affirmations, either aloud or silently, believing in their truth.)
"I am worthy of all my desires and dreams."
"Abundance flows to me effortlessly and easily."
"I trust the process of manifestation, and I am open to receiving."
"I am a magnet for love, success, and prosperity."

5. Gratitude Practice
(Take a moment to express gratitude for what you already have and for what is coming.)
"Thank you, Universe, for the blessings in my life."
"I am grateful for the opportunities that align with my desires."
"Thank you for supporting me on this journey of manifestation."

6. Action Steps
(Identify actionable steps you can take this week to support your manifestation.)
What will I do this week to move closer to my desires?

BUTTERFLY SPIRIT
CHECK OUT ALL MY BOOKS!

BUTTERFLY SPIRIT

✿ Nature Connection Prayer Page ✿

Date: ____________________________

🖋 Nature Prayers for Transformation:
Write your own nature-inspired prayer for growth and abundance:

☑ Check off when practiced in nature:
Meditated in a natural setting.
Said my prayer outdoors.
Observed nature's beauty and abundance.

BUTTERFLY SPIRIT

Celebrating Small Wins Page

Date: ________________________

Today's Achievements:
List your wins, big or small:

____

____

____

Celebration Actions:

What will I do to celebrate my progress?

____

____

Empowering Affirmations:
Create affirmations to replace limiting beliefs:
I am worthy of abundance.

____

____

BUTTERFLY SPIRIT

🌈 Abundance Mindset Reflections 🌈
Date: _______________________________
⚓ Limiting Beliefs to Release:
What beliefs do I want to let go of?

💜 Gratitude Checklist 💜
Date: _______________________________
🌸 Today, I am grateful for:
List five things you appreciate today.

Gratitude Actions:
Check all that apply today!
I expressed gratitude to someone.
I wrote in my gratitude journal.
I shared my appreciation on social media.
I did something kind for myself.
I acknowledged a personal achievement.

BUTTERFLY SPIRIT

⚘ Transformation Goals Page ⚘
Date: _______________________________
My Transformation Intentions:
What changes do I want to embrace?

Visualizing My Abundance:
Picture what success looks like for you:

BUTTERFLY SPIRIT

🦋 Inspired Action Checklist 🦋

Date: _________________________

Actions to Attract Abundance:
What steps will I take today?

Networking Opportunities:
Individuals to connect with:

✓ Check off actions taken:

☐ Reached out to someone.

☐ Attended a networking event.

☐ Engaged in a community project.

BUTTERFLY SPIRIT

Here's a refined set of fill-in-the-blank, checklist grid journal pages that emphasize beauty and detail, incorporating the butterfly spirit theme.

These pages are designed to be functional yet visually appealing, encouraging a joyful journaling experience.

Butterfly Spirit Journal Pages
🦋 Transformation Goals Page 🦋
Date: _______________________
My Transformation Intentions:
What changes do I want to embrace?

Visualizing My Abundance:
Picture what success looks like for you:

💜 Gratitude Checklist 💜

Date: _______________________
Today, I am grateful for:
List five things you appreciate today.

Gratitude Actions:
Check all that apply today!
I expressed gratitude to someone.
I wrote in my gratitude journal.
I shared my appreciation on social media.
I did something kind for myself.
I acknowledged a personal achievement.

BUTTERFLY SPIRIT

Weekly Manifestation Script
Preparation
Find a quiet space and take a few deep breaths to center yourself.
1. Opening Invocation
"Dear Universe, I open my heart and mind to receive the blessings of my desires. I trust in the process of manifestation."
2. Reflection on Desires
This week, I desire:

----

3. Visualization
(Close your eyes and visualize your desires as already achieved.)
Feel the joy and gratitude as if they are yours now.
4. Affirmations
"I am worthy of my desires."
"Abundance flows to me effortlessly."
"I trust the timing of my manifestations."
5. Gratitude
"Thank you, Universe, for all my blessings and for the desires that are on their way to me."
6. Action Steps
This week, I will:

----

7. Closing Intention
"I trust that my desires are manifesting in perfect timing. So it is, and so it shall be."

BUTTERFLY SPIRIT

Weekly Manifestation Ritual Script
Preparation
Find a quiet space where you can sit comfortably without distractions.
Gather items that resonate with you (e.g., crystals, candles, or meaningful objects).
Take a few deep breaths to center yourself.
1. Opening Invocation
(Speak or write this aloud)
"Dear Universe, God, and my higher self, I come to you with an open heart and mind. I acknowledge the power of my intentions and the beauty of my desires. I am grateful for this moment to align with my true self and manifest my dreams."
2. Reflection on Desires
(Take a moment to reflect on the following questions. You can write your responses in a journal.)
What are my desires this week?

Why are these desires important to me?

BUTTERFLY SPIRIT

3. Visualization
(Close your eyes and visualize your desires as if they have already manifested.)
Imagine how it feels to achieve each desire.
Engage all your senses—what do you see, hear, feel, and smell?
Spend 5-10 minutes in this visualization, allowing the feelings of joy and fulfillment to wash over you.

4. Affirmations
(Repeat the following affirmations, either aloud or silently, believing in their truth.)
"I am worthy of all my desires and dreams."
"Abundance flows to me effortlessly and easily."
"I trust the process of manifestation, and I am open to receiving."
"I am a magnet for love, success, and prosperity."

5. Gratitude Practice
(Take a moment to express gratitude for what you already have and for what is coming.)
"Thank you, Universe, for the blessings in my life."
"I am grateful for the opportunities that align with my desires."
"Thank you for supporting me on this journey of manifestation."

6. Action Steps
(Identify actionable steps you can take this week to support your manifestation.)
What will I do this week to move closer to my desires?

BUTTERFLY SPIRIT
CHECK OUT ALL MY BOOKS!

BUTTERFLY SPIRIT

🌿 Nature Connection Prayer Page 🌿

Date: _______________________________

🌙 Nature Prayers for Transformation:
Write your own nature-inspired prayer for growth and abundance:

____

____

☑ Check off when practiced in nature:
Meditated in a natural setting.
Said my prayer outdoors.
Observed nature's beauty and abundance.

BUTTERFLY SPIRIT

Celebrating Small Wins Page

Date: ___________________________

Today's Achievements:
List your wins, big or small:

Celebration Actions:

What will I do to celebrate my progress?

Empowering Affirmations:
Create affirmations to replace limiting beliefs:
I am worthy of abundance.

BUTTERFLY SPIRIT

🌈 Abundance Mindset Reflections 🌈
Date: ________________________
⚓ Limiting Beliefs to Release:
What beliefs do I want to let go of?

🖤 Gratitude Checklist 🖤
Date: ________________________
🌼 Today, I am grateful for:
List five things you appreciate today.

Gratitude Actions:
Check all that apply today!
I expressed gratitude to someone.
I wrote in my gratitude journal.
I shared my appreciation on social media.
I did something kind for myself.
I acknowledged a personal achievement.

BUTTERFLY SPIRIT

⚘ Transformation Goals Page ⚘
Date: _________________________________
My Transformation Intentions:
What changes do I want to embrace?

⚘ Visualizing My Abundance:
Picture what success looks like for you:

BUTTERFLY SPIRIT

🦋 Inspired Action Checklist 🦋

Date: _______________________

Actions to Attract Abundance:
What steps will I take today?

Networking Opportunities:
Individuals to connect with:

✓ Check off actions taken:

☐ Reached out to someone.

☐ Attended a networking event.

☐ Engaged in a community project.

BUTTERFLY SPIRIT

Here's a refined set of fill-in-the-blank, checklist grid journal pages that emphasize beauty and detail, incorporating the butterfly spirit theme.

These pages are designed to be functional yet visually appealing, encouraging a joyful journaling experience.

Butterfly Spirit Journal Pages
🦋 Transformation Goals Page 🦋
Date: _______________________
My Transformation Intentions:
What changes do I want to embrace?

Visualizing My Abundance:
Picture what success looks like for you:

🖤 Gratitude Checklist 🖤

Date: _______________________
Today, I am grateful for:
List five things you appreciate today.

Gratitude Actions:
Check all that apply today!
I expressed gratitude to someone.
I wrote in my gratitude journal.
I shared my appreciation on social media.
I did something kind for myself.
I acknowledged a personal achievement.

BUTTERFLY SPIRIT

Weekly Manifestation Script
Preparation
Find a quiet space and take a few deep breaths to center yourself.
1. Opening Invocation
"Dear Universe, I open my heart and mind to receive the blessings of my desires. I trust in the process of manifestation."
2. Reflection on Desires
This week, I desire:

____
____
____

3. Visualization
(Close your eyes and visualize your desires as already achieved.)
Feel the joy and gratitude as if they are yours now.
4. Affirmations
"I am worthy of my desires."
"Abundance flows to me effortlessly."
"I trust the timing of my manifestations."
5. Gratitude
"Thank you, Universe, for all my blessings and for the desires that are on their way to me."
6. Action Steps
This week, I will:

____
____
____

7. Closing Intention
"I trust that my desires are manifesting in perfect timing. So it is, and so it shall be."

BUTTERFLY SPIRIT

Weekly Manifestation Ritual Script
Preparation
Find a quiet space where you can sit comfortably without distractions.
Gather items that resonate with you (e.g., crystals, candles, or meaningful objects).
Take a few deep breaths to center yourself.
1. Opening Invocation
(Speak or write this aloud)
"Dear Universe, God, and my higher self, I come to you with an open heart and mind. I acknowledge the power of my intentions and the beauty of my desires. I am grateful for this moment to align with my true self and manifest my dreams."
2. Reflection on Desires
(Take a moment to reflect on the following questions. You can write your responses in a journal.)
What are my desires this week?

Why are these desires important to me?

BUTTERFLY SPIRIT

3. Visualization
(Close your eyes and visualize your desires as if they have already manifested.)
Imagine how it feels to achieve each desire.
Engage all your senses—what do you see, hear, feel, and smell?
Spend 5-10 minutes in this visualization, allowing the feelings of joy and fulfillment to wash over you.

4. Affirmations
(Repeat the following affirmations, either aloud or silently, believing in their truth.)
"I am worthy of all my desires and dreams."
"Abundance flows to me effortlessly and easily."
"I trust the process of manifestation, and I am open to receiving."
"I am a magnet for love, success, and prosperity."

5. Gratitude Practice
(Take a moment to express gratitude for what you already have and for what is coming.)
"Thank you, Universe, for the blessings in my life."
"I am grateful for the opportunities that align with my desires."
"Thank you for supporting me on this journey of manifestation."

6. Action Steps
(Identify actionable steps you can take this week to support your manifestation.)
What will I do this week to move closer to my desires?

____

____

____

BUTTERFLY SPIRIT
CHECK OUT ALL MY BOOKS!

BUTTERFLY SPIRIT

✿ Nature Connection Prayer Page ✿

Date: ________________________________

🪶 Nature Prayers for Transformation:

Write your own nature-inspired prayer for growth and abundance:

____

____

☑ Check off when practiced in nature:

Meditated in a natural setting.

Said my prayer outdoors.

Observed nature's beauty and abundance.

BUTTERFLY SPIRIT

Celebrating Small Wins Page

Date: _______________________

Today's Achievements:
List your wins, big or small:

____

____

____

Celebration Actions:

What will I do to celebrate my progress?

____

____

Empowering Affirmations:
Create affirmations to replace limiting beliefs:
I am worthy of abundance.

____

____

BUTTERFLY SPIRIT

🌈 Abundance Mindset Reflections 🌈
Date: ____________________________

☻ Limiting Beliefs to Release:
What beliefs do I want to let go of?

💜 Gratitude Checklist 💜
Date: ____________________________

☀ Today, I am grateful for:
List five things you appreciate today.

⬇ Gratitude Actions:
Check all that apply today!
I expressed gratitude to someone.
I wrote in my gratitude journal.
I shared my appreciation on social media.
I did something kind for myself.
I acknowledged a personal achievement.

BUTTERFLY SPIRIT

🦋 Transformation Goals Page 🦋
Date: ________________________________
My Transformation Intentions:
What changes do I want to embrace?

Visualizing My Abundance:
Picture what success looks like for you:

BUTTERFLY SPIRIT

🦋 Inspired Action Checklist 🦋

Date: _______________________________

Actions to Attract Abundance:
What steps will I take today?

____

____

____

Networking Opportunities:
Individuals to connect with:

____

____

✓ Check off actions taken:

☐ Reached out to someone.

☐ Attended a networking event.

☐ Engaged in a community project.

BUTTERFLY SPIRIT

Here's a refined set of fill-in-the-blank, checklist grid journal pages that emphasize beauty and detail, incorporating the butterfly spirit theme.

These pages are designed to be functional yet visually appealing, encouraging a joyful journaling experience.

Butterfly Spirit Journal Pages
🦋 Transformation Goals Page 🦋
Date: _______________________
My Transformation Intentions:
What changes do I want to embrace?

Visualizing My Abundance:
Picture what success looks like for you:

💜 Gratitude Checklist 💜

Date: _______________________
Today, I am grateful for:
List five things you appreciate today.

Gratitude Actions:
Check all that apply today!
I expressed gratitude to someone.
I wrote in my gratitude journal.
I shared my appreciation on social media.
I did something kind for myself.
I acknowledged a personal achievement.

BUTTERFLY SPIRIT

Weekly Manifestation Script
Preparation
Find a quiet space and take a few deep breaths to center yourself.
1. Opening Invocation
"Dear Universe, I open my heart and mind to receive the blessings of my
desires. I trust in the process of manifestation."
2. Reflection on Desires
This week, I desire:

----
3. Visualization
(Close your eyes and visualize your desires as already achieved.)
Feel the joy and gratitude as if they are yours now.
4. Affirmations
"I am worthy of my desires."
"Abundance flows to me effortlessly."
"I trust the timing of my manifestations."
5. Gratitude
"Thank you, Universe, for all my blessings and for the desires that are on
their way to me."
6. Action Steps
This week, I will:

----
7. Closing Intention
"I trust that my desires are manifesting in perfect timing. So it is, and so it
shall be."

BUTTERFLY SPIRIT

Weekly Manifestation Ritual Script
Preparation
Find a quiet space where you can sit comfortably without distractions.
Gather items that resonate with you (e.g., crystals, candles, or meaningful objects).
Take a few deep breaths to center yourself.
1. Opening Invocation
(Speak or write this aloud)
"Dear Universe, God, and my higher self, I come to you with an open heart and mind. I acknowledge the power of my intentions and the beauty of my desires. I am grateful for this moment to align with my true self and manifest my dreams."
2. Reflection on Desires
(Take a moment to reflect on the following questions. You can write your responses in a journal.)
What are my desires this week?

Why are these desires important to me?

BUTTERFLY SPIRIT

3. Visualization
(Close your eyes and visualize your desires as if they have already manifested.)
Imagine how it feels to achieve each desire.
Engage all your senses—what do you see, hear, feel, and smell?
Spend 5-10 minutes in this visualization, allowing the feelings of joy and fulfillment to wash over you.

4. Affirmations
(Repeat the following affirmations, either aloud or silently, believing in their truth.)
"I am worthy of all my desires and dreams."
"Abundance flows to me effortlessly and easily."
"I trust the process of manifestation, and I am open to receiving."
"I am a magnet for love, success, and prosperity."

5. Gratitude Practice
(Take a moment to express gratitude for what you already have and for what is coming.)
"Thank you, Universe, for the blessings in my life."
"I am grateful for the opportunities that align with my desires."
"Thank you for supporting me on this journey of manifestation."

6. Action Steps
(Identify actionable steps you can take this week to support your manifestation.)
What will I do this week to move closer to my desires?

BUTTERFLY SPIRIT
CHECK OUT ALL MY BOOKS!

BUTTERFLY SPIRIT

❧ Nature Connection Prayer Page ❧

Date: ____________________________

Nature Prayers for Transformation:
Write your own nature-inspired prayer for growth and abundance:

____

____

☑ Check off when practiced in nature:
Meditated in a natural setting.
Said my prayer outdoors.
Observed nature's beauty and abundance.

BUTTERFLY SPIRIT

Celebrating Small Wins Page

Date: _______________________

✦ Today's Achievements:
List your wins, big or small:

Celebration Actions:

What will I do to celebrate my progress?

Empowering Affirmations:
Create affirmations to replace limiting beliefs:
I am worthy of abundance.

BUTTERFLY SPIRIT

🌈 Abundance Mindset Reflections 🌈
Date: _______________________________
🌸 Limiting Beliefs to Release:
What beliefs do I want to let go of?

💗 Gratitude Checklist 💗
Date: _______________________________
🌼 Today, I am grateful for:
List five things you appreciate today.

Gratitude Actions:
Check all that apply today!
I expressed gratitude to someone.
I wrote in my gratitude journal.
I shared my appreciation on social media.
I did something kind for myself.
I acknowledged a personal achievement.

BUTTERFLY SPIRIT

🦋 Transformation Goals Page 🦋
Date: ______________________________
My Transformation Intentions:
What changes do I want to embrace?

Visualizing My Abundance:
Picture what success looks like for you:

BUTTERFLY SPIRIT

🦋 Inspired Action Checklist 🦋

Date: ________________________

Actions to Attract Abundance:
What steps will I take today?

Networking Opportunities:
Individuals to connect with:

✓ Check off actions taken:

☐ Reached out to someone.

☐ Attended a networking event.

☐ Engaged in a community project.

BUTTERFLY SPIRIT

Here's a refined set of *fill-in-the-blank*, checklist grid journal pages that emphasize beauty and detail, incorporating the butterfly spirit theme.

These pages are designed to be functional yet visually appealing, encouraging a joyful journaling experience.

Butterfly Spirit Journal Pages
❀ Transformation Goals Page ❀
Date: ______________________________
My Transformation Intentions:
What changes do I want to embrace?

Visualizing My Abundance:
Picture what success looks like for you:

Gratitude Checklist

Date: ______________________________
Today, I am grateful for:
List five things you appreciate today.

Gratitude Actions:
Check all that apply today!
I expressed gratitude to someone.
I wrote in my gratitude journal.
I shared my appreciation on social media.
I did something kind for myself.
I acknowledged a personal achievement.

BUTTERFLY SPIRIT

Weekly Manifestation Script
Preparation
Find a quiet space and take a few deep breaths to center yourself.
1. Opening Invocation
"Dear Universe, I open my heart and mind to receive the blessings of my desires. I trust in the process of manifestation."
2. Reflection on Desires
This week, I desire:

____

____

____

3. Visualization
(Close your eyes and visualize your desires as already achieved.)
Feel the joy and gratitude as if they are yours now.
4. Affirmations
"I am worthy of my desires."
"Abundance flows to me effortlessly."
"I trust the timing of my manifestations."
5. Gratitude
"Thank you, Universe, for all my blessings and for the desires that are on their way to me."
6. Action Steps
This week, I will:

____

____

____

7. Closing Intention
"I trust that my desires are manifesting in perfect timing. So it is, and so it shall be."

BUTTERFLY SPIRIT

Weekly Manifestation Ritual Script
Preparation
Find a quiet space where you can sit comfortably without distractions.
Gather items that resonate with you (e.g., crystals, candles, or meaningful objects).
Take a few deep breaths to center yourself.
1. Opening Invocation
(Speak or write this aloud)
"Dear Universe, God, and my higher self, I come to you with an open heart and mind. I acknowledge the power of my intentions and the beauty of my desires. I am grateful for this moment to align with my true self and manifest my dreams."
2. Reflection on Desires
(Take a moment to reflect on the following questions. You can write your responses in a journal.)
What are my desires this week?

Why are these desires important to me?

BUTTERFLY SPIRIT

3. Visualization
(Close your eyes and visualize your desires as if they have already manifested.)
Imagine how it feels to achieve each desire.
Engage all your senses—what do you see, hear, feel, and smell?
Spend 5-10 minutes in this visualization, allowing the feelings of joy and fulfillment to wash over you.

4. Affirmations
(Repeat the following affirmations, either aloud or silently, believing in their truth.)
"I am worthy of all my desires and dreams."
"Abundance flows to me effortlessly and easily."
"I trust the process of manifestation, and I am open to receiving."
"I am a magnet for love, success, and prosperity."

5. Gratitude Practice
(Take a moment to express gratitude for what you already have and for what is coming.)
"Thank you, Universe, for the blessings in my life."
"I am grateful for the opportunities that align with my desires."
"Thank you for supporting me on this journey of manifestation."

6. Action Steps
(Identify actionable steps you can take this week to support your manifestation.)
What will I do this week to move closer to my desires?

____

____

____

BUTTERFLY SPIRIT

Disclaimer

The information provided in BUTTERFLY SPIRIT is for educational and informational purposes only. The author does not intend for this book to serve as a substitute for professional advice or guidance. Readers should consult with a qualified professional for any personal, financial, medical, or psychological issues.

The practices and exercises described in this book are based on personal experiences and research. Individual results may vary. By reading this book, you acknowledge that you are responsible for your own actions and decisions. The author shall not be liable for any direct or indirect damages resulting from the use or misuse of the information contained herein.

BUTTERFLY SPIRIT

Conclusion

As you reach the end of BUTTERFLY SPIRIT, I hope you feel empowered and inspired to embrace your transformation. Remember, the journey does not stop here; it continues with every decision you make, every belief you nurture, and every action you take.

Your Butterfly Spirit has the power to rise above challenges and manifest the life you desire.

Take the insights and practices shared in this book and integrate them into your daily life. Continue to reflect, visualize, and affirm your worthiness. Trust that the universe is conspiring in your favor and that your dreams are within reach.

Thank you for allowing me to be a part of your journey. May you always fly high, embracing the beauty of your transformation and the abundance that awaits you.

BUTTERFLY SPIRIT THOUGHTS

BUTTERFLY SPIRIT THOUGHTS

BUTTERFLY SPIRIT

BUTTERFLY SPIRIT THOUGHTS

BUTTERFLY SPIRIT
THOUGHTS

BUTTERFLY SPIRIT THOUGHTS

BUTTERFLY SPIRIT THOUGHTS

BUTTERFLY SPIRIT THOUGHTS

BUTTERFLY SPIRIT
THOUGHTS

BUTTERFLY SPIRIT THOUGHTS

BUTTERFLY SPIRIT THOUGHTS

BUTTERFLY SPIRIT THOUGHTS

BUTTERFLY SPIRIT THOUGHTS

BUTTERFLY SPIRIT THOUGHTS

BUTTERFLY SPIRIT THOUGHTS

BUTTERFLY SPIRIT THOUGHTS

BUTTERFLY SPIRIT
THOUGHTS

BUTTERFLY SPIRIT THOUGHTS

BUTTERFLY SPIRIT THOUGHTS

BUTTERFLY SPIRIT THOUGHTS

BUTTERFLY SPIRIT THOUGHTS

BUTTERFLY SPIRIT

BUTTERFLY SPIRIT THOUGHTS

BUTTERFLY SPIRIT THOUGHTS

BUTTERFLY SPIRIT THOUGHTS

BUTTERFLY SPIRIT THOUGHTS

BUTTERFLY SPIRIT THOUGHTS

BUTTERFLY SPIRIT
THOUGHTS

BUTTERFLY SPIRIT THOUGHTS

BUTTERFLY SPIRIT
THOUGHTS

BUTTERFLY SPIRIT THOUGHTS

BUTTERFLY SPIRIT THOUGHTS

BUTTERFLY SPIRIT THOUGHTS

BUTTERFLY SPIRIT
THOUGHTS

BUTTERFLY SPIRIT THOUGHTS

BUTTERFLY SPIRIT
THOUGHTS

BUTTERFLY SPIRIT THOUGHTS

BUTTERFLY SPIRIT THOUGHTS

BUTTERFLY SPIRIT THOUGHTS

BUTTERFLY SPIRIT THOUGHTS

BUTTERFLY SPIRIT THOUGHTS

BUTTERFLY SPIRIT
THOUGHTS